"This is an important book that provides a realistic, powerful, and sen for individual clients and tailor a unique treatment for each one. Focusing on specific processes within, Hofmann, Hayes, and Lorscheid direct us to the best ideas from a range of approaches. A wonderful tool-box and conceptual road map for the clinician. This is the voice of modern cognitive behavioral therapy (CBT), and it rings clear."

> —**Robert L. Leahy, PhD**, director at the American Institute for Cognitive Therapy, and
> author of *Emotional Schema Therapy*

"Process-based therapy (PBT) is a comprehensive and innovative model that brings best practices to life. Intelligently written in a series of practical steps, it will advance clinical applications regardless of one's level of experience or theoretical predilection."

> —**Jeffrey K. Zeig, PhD**, founder and CEO of The Milton H Erickson Foundation, and
> architect of The Evolution of Psychotherapy Conference

"Our many distinct therapeutic approaches can be deeply enhanced by the wisdom and practical tools in this timely and important work. Exploring how human beings live within networks of systems, our articu-late and thoughtful guides illuminate how an evidence-based approach can be tailored to the individual and the empirically validated processes of change to deepen and strengthen how we help not only reduce suffering, but bring lasting change to those for whom we care. Harnessing research-based knowledge of the embodied and relational human mind and how it both gets stuck in patterns of dysfunction as well as liber-ated with transformation, this book will be of benefit to anyone helping the development of individuals across the life span."

> —**Daniel J. Siegel, MD**, *New York Times* bestselling author of *Mind*, *Aware*,
> *The Mindful Therapist*, *Mindsight*, and *The Developing Mind*

"With any science, it is often imperative to take a step back, evaluate its progress, and identify bold new future directions. That is exactly what Hofmann, Hayes, and Lorscheid have done with this book. By focusing on processes, rather than content, they articulate a unique way of suggesting, investigating, and implementing effective approaches to best help people reach important life goals. This volume is an impor-tant step forward!"

> —**Arthur M. Nezu, PhD, DHL, ABPP**, distinguished professor of psychological
> and brain sciences at Drexel University, and editor in chief of *Clinical Psychology*

"This text does an exemplary job linking processes and treatments, and includes many clinical scenarios that will greatly aid graduate students who are mastering acceptance and commitment therapy (ACT) concepts. I greatly appreciate the incorporation of the evolutionary science (ES) concepts into the meta-model described in the text for predicting and influencing both adaptive and maladaptive behaviors. This is a highly pragmatic approach to delivering PBT."

> —**Ruth Anne Rehfeldt, PhD, BCBA-D**, chair of the bachelor's program in psychology,
> and professor of applied behavior analysis at the Chicago School of Professional Psychology

"This book shines a light on an important aspect of treatment: the transdiagnostic processes that lead to dysfunction and that should be targeted in therapy. The authors present a system for identifying and modifying these critical processes."

—**Judith S. Beck, PhD**, president of the Beck Institute for Cognitive Behavior Therapy, and author of *Cognitive Behavior Therapy*

"Each day, another trademarked intervention package appears on the market. I don't want a new package and new jargon. Thank goodness for this book. It provides a clear and systematic way to understand effective processes that occur across different packages. It's got me thinking differently about client suffering, in terms of dynamic systems, rather than static 'things.' The book is so practical and easy to understand. I love it."

—**Joseph Ciarrochi, PhD**, research professor at Australian Catholic University, and coauthor of *Your Life, Your Way*; *The Thriving Adolescent*; and *The Weight Escape*

"Something important is missing from evidence-based psychological treatments and the research supporting these interventions—a clear and essential focus on the individual receiving the treatment. The authors, who are among the most distinguished clinical scientists in the world, attack this problem head-on with PBT. In this manual, clinicians will learn to refocus powerful principles of psychological change on the individuals being treated. Every clinician should be familiar with these strategies."

—**David H. Barlow PhD, ABPP**, professor of psychology and psychiatry emeritus, and founder of the Center for Anxiety and Related Disorders (CARD)

"This book is a breath of fresh air. It calls it like it is. The differential treatment model of what treatment for what disorder has had its day. Their proposed process-based approach to treatment moves us forward to a promising new transdiagnostic, transtheoretical approach focused on evidence-based processes of change that fit the needs of a given client. This is the future. A must-read, wonderful contribution."

—**Leslie Greenberg, PhD**, distinguished research professor emeritus of psychology at York University, author of *Changing Emotion with Emotion*, and coeditor of *Patterns of Change*

"I love the idiographic approach to psychotherapy this book describes! PBT offers the clinician a welcome alternative to treatment guided by disorder-focused protocols. This book teaches the therapist to build a model of the individual case, and to use the model to guide treatment—monitoring progress and making adjustments based on the progress-monitoring data as the therapy proceeds. The intellectual framework for the model is mind-expanding and groundbreaking."

—**Jacqueline B. Persons**, director of the Oakland CBT Center; clinical professor at the University of California, Berkeley; and author of *The Case Formulation Approach to Cognitive-Behavior Therapy*

Learning Process-Based Therapy

A Skills Training Manual for Targeting the Core Processes of Psychological Change in Clinical Practice

Stefan G. Hofmann, PhD
Steven C. Hayes, PhD
David N. Lorscheid

CONTEXT PRESS
An Imprint of New Harbinger Publications, Inc.

Publisher's Note

This publication is designed to provide accurate and authoritative information in regard to the subject matter covered. It is sold with the understanding that the publisher is not engaged in rendering psychological, financial, legal, or other professional services. If expert assistance or counseling is needed, the services of a competent professional should be sought.

Distributed in Canada by Raincoast Books

NEW HARBINGER PUBLICATIONS is a
registered trademark of New Harbinger Publications, Inc.

Copyright © 2021 by Stefan G. Hofmann, Steven C. Hayes, and David N. Lorscheid
Context Press
An imprint of New Harbinger Publications, Inc.
5674 Shattuck Avenue
Oakland, CA 94609
www.newharbinger.com

Figure 9.6 is copyright Stefan G. Hofmann

Cover design by Sara Christain; Acquired by Catharine Sutker; Edited by Rona Bernstein

Library of Congress Cataloging-in-Publication Data on file

Names: Hofmann, Stefan G., author. | Hayes, Steven C., author. | Lorscheid, David N., author.
Title: Learning process-based therapy : a skills training manual for targeting the core processes of
   psychological change in clinical practice / Stefan G. Hofmann, Ph.D, Steven C. Hayes, Ph.D,
   David N. Lorscheid.
Identifiers: LCCN 2021027778 | ISBN 9781684037551 (trade paperback)
Subjects: LCSH: Psychotherapy. | Evidence-based medicine. | Medicine--Decision making. |
   Psychotherapist and patient.
Classification: LCC RC475 .H64 2021 | DDC 616.89/14--dc23
LC record available at https://lccn.loc.gov/2021027778

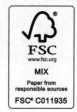

Printed in the United States of America

24   23   22

10   9   8   7   6   5   4   3

Contents

Prologue

For decades, mental and behavioral health practitioners have been told in their graduate training programs that their work needs to be "evidence-based." They learn to read the scientific literature. They are carefully schooled in "diagnoses." They learn evidence-based protocols. They acquire statistical skills.

But something is wrong. Effect sizes are not rising. The prevalence of problems in mental and behavioral health is not falling. Evidence-based care is far too uncommon. Too many practitioners find this model of evidence-based care to be stultifying. And the field itself is progressing far too slowly.

We believe that what we are seeing is the end of an era—and the beginning of a new one. Evidence-based care came to be defined as the delivery of empirically tested protocols targeting psychiatric syndromes. The biomedicalization of human suffering on which this model stood did not pay off in the way that promoters had hoped. Protocols proliferated and fit the needs of individuals poorly.

It's time for something fundamentally different.

Process-based therapy (PBT) is a new definition of what evidence-based therapy even means. It's not a new treatment method—it's a new way of thinking about treatment methods. We believe that by taking a far more idiographic approach and learning a new form of functional analysis based on processes of change, the field can move forward. This new approach links evidence-based processes to evidence-based treatment kernels, organized into more parsimonious and yet more comprehensive models that will better address what clients really want.

In this book we provide a robust set of skills and tools for learning this new approach that builds on the best of our clinical traditions and on the solid core of intervention science.

It's time for something fundamentally different. If you are ready to begin, so are we.

Stefan G. Hofmann

Steven C. Hayes

David N. Lorscheid

CHAPTER 1

Rethinking Clinical Science and Practice

Bill, a thirty-year-old man, pursues treatment after a recent breakup from his girlfriend. He is feeling depressed. The breakup led him to ruminate more often, which only lowered his mood even more. Sara is an empathic young therapist who just completed her internship, where she studied a popular cognitive behavioral therapy (CBT) protocol to treat depression. She skillfully conducted each session according to a structured treatment manual for depression. After conducting an initial assessment and providing psychoeducation, she introduced the three-component model of mood, describing its cognitive, emotional, and biophysiological dimensions. She administered monitoring forms to track Bill's behaviors, thoughts, and feelings, and then went on to focus on his dysfunctional thoughts and maladaptive behaviors. Sara particularly targeted Bill's ruminative tendencies, as was described in the therapy manual.

After twelve sessions, Sara assessed Bill's depression using the Beck Depression Inventory (BDI), which showed a moderate but notable decline, and both were fairly satisfied with the outcome. Based on Bill's improvement, he might even have been considered a "responder" if he had been part of a clinical trial. After Sara reached the last session of the protocol, she decided that it was time to stop the treatment. She sent Bill home with the instruction to keep practicing the skills he learned during treatment, including his behavioral activation exercises and the skills to target rumination and other cognitive errors.

When Bill left Sara's office, he thanked her. On his way home, however, he felt a sense of uneasiness. He felt less depressed than before, but he realized that he was not close to where he wanted to be emotionally and in general with his life. He still felt lonely and disconnected after the breakup. He waived it off with the thought that therapy can't do everything, and perhaps he was just not the kind of person who can have committed relationships. The feeling of unease remained, and he wondered what he would do now.

Sara felt good about her case. She followed a well-validated treatment protocol for depression, and she thought that she did a fine job with it. Based on traditional outcome measures, the case was clearly successful, and she chalked it up that way. Her attention soon moved on to other cases and clients, and Bill gradually slid into memory.

Sara would never find out that Bill was feeling uneasy and vulnerable even as he left his last session. She would never learn that in a few months, his loneliness would become an all-encompassing focus, and he would slip back into depression, even having suicidal thoughts.

What might have gone wrong? We cannot be sure that all of Bill's issues could have been addressed successfully, but we can be sure that several of them were not really addressed at all. Sara did not target some aspects of Bill's problems—such as his loneliness, his relationships, and his feeling of social isolation and unhappiness. Bill often thought about these issues and was wondering where they came from and what maintained them. Sara touched on these issues only briefly and thought they would resolve naturally after she had targeted Bill's tendency to ruminate and his depressed mood and actions. Relationship skills were not a notable part of the structured treatment manual, which she knew so well. Since she had successfully treated the depression with an evidence-based set of methods, she believed that would be enough.

Except, it wasn't.

THE PROTOCOLS-FOR-SYNDROMES GAME

Does Bill have a disease called depression? And how can it be defined? It sounds like an obvious and easily answered question, but it isn't. COVID-19 is a virus that caused a worldwide pandemic. We are in the midst of it as we are writing these words. Many people have died because of the virus. Others who were infected had barely any symptoms, some none at all. Measuring one's body temperature is a quick way to identify those who might have the virus, but it misses many. A much more accurate test is to look for antibodies, or for the RNA fragments of the virus itself. The presence of those biological markers clearly defines the disease.

There is no such test for depression or anxiety or schizophrenia or any other psychological disorder. Not one. And there is no vaccine that immunizes people from getting a particular mental disorder. Yet, for decades, psychiatry has been holding on to a medical illness model that assumes that symptoms of a psychological disorder are the expressions of an underlying disease. The *Diagnostic and Statistical Manual of Mental Disorders* (DSM) and the *International Classification of Diseases* (ICD) are tools to achieve that end. Earlier versions of the DSM and ICD were based on psychoanalytic theory and assumed that mental disorders are the result of deep-seated conflicts. Modern versions point to dysfunctions in biological, psychological, and developmental processes as the primary cause. Above all, over the last forty years, academic psychiatry has been hoping to identify biological markers for mental disorders, for instance in genes or in brain circuits.

This quest remains unsuccessful, and as scientific knowledge has increased, this long hoped for outcome has slid even further into the distance. For example, full genomic analyses of nearly half a million people have failed to support the relevance of any of the frequently studied genes for common psychiatric disorders (e.g., Border et al., 2019). It appears that genetic factors can interact with each other and with a person's history and context to produce mental struggles many, many different ways.

This lack of success has not led to the abandonment of the latent disease model. Arguably the most popular idea has been that mental disorders are caused by some imbalance of neurotransmitters. Therefore, drug companies developed, tested, and marketed drugs to alter this neurotransmitter system, especially serotonin, dopamine, GABA, and glutamate. These drugs were tested in randomized placebo-controlled trials. Some of these studies reported some modest effect on some of the symptoms of the presumed disorder (but many other studies did not). Some bold and innovative psychological researchers began to compare the efficacy of those drugs to psychological interventions, primarily CBT but also some other forms of evidence-based treatment. In order to keep the psychological treatments symptom focused and to adequately conduct these trials, treatment protocols had to be developed.

The results shook the field. Often published in high-level psychiatry journals, they frequently generated a lot of controversy. The good news was that these trials often found that CBT in particular was as good as or even better than the most effective pharmacological drugs. The bad news, however, was that CBT began losing its theoretical foundation and became a symptom-focused, protocol-based intervention targeting the disorder rather than treating the client. Today, CBT is considered a mainstream, gold-standard psychological treatment, acknowledged and recognized by even the most biologically oriented psychiatrist.

The scientific and social cost of this achievement was high. Despite the wealth of knowledge gathered from clinical trials and meta-analyses of the various forms of evidence-based therapy, outcome results did little by way of explaining important individual differences in presentation and treatment response, or in fostering an understanding of the mechanisms of treatment change, especially when differences of these kinds were averaged across groups. A randomized clinical trial comparing the depression levels of participants across various interventions using a central outcome measure (e.g., Clinical Global Impression scale) treats between-participant variability in responding merely as an estimate of extraneous factors and measurement error. Consequently, information is lost about the unique pattern of improvement or deterioration of the individual and its relation to presentation, context, and treatment. Much of this research involves investigating the likelihood that treatment will work for a diagnosis rather than for the processes, circumstances, and symptoms that characterize the individual.

Meanwhile, an entire generation has grown up with the commercially useful but scientifically false idea that experiencing mental struggles means you have a specific biologically based brain dysfunction. As a result, consumers are less interested in psychotherapy, regardless of what the data suggest. From 1998 to 2007 (the most recent decade with good numbers), the number of people using only psychological change methods fell nearly 50 percent, while the number of those using psychological approaches along with medications fell about 30 percent. What soared was the use of medication alone—nearly two out of three people with psychological struggles now receive *only* medications as interventions (Olfson & Marcus, 2010).

Ultimate success of the "protocols-for-syndromes" game depended on identifying functional disease entities, or at least seeing highly specific treatment effects organized by syndromes. When neither appeared, the scientific path toward a mature form of evidence-based therapy turned into a brute force empiricism in which almost everything should be compared to almost everything else in a wide variety of syndromes or subsyndromes. The mathematics of this research approach makes it impossible to mount, even if the number of new intervention methods and syndromal entities could magically be held to its current number—which it cannot.

The protocols-for-syndromes era had a coherent set of key assumptions built into its scientific and public health strategy—but every one of them is now being openly challenged and some are now known to be false. At the same time, a powerful alternative strategic agenda is emerging that echoes some of the process-based and idiographic assumptions of the earliest days of behavioral research, as well as the therapy based upon it.

This alternative agenda has taken time to become fully visible due to the other undesirable effects of the latent disease model. For one thing, this model tended to blind treatment developers to the role of normal psychological processes in behavioral outcomes. Furthermore, it neglected clients' preferences for pragmatic outcomes, and instead prioritized the preferred list of signs and symptoms. It reduced human suffering to hypothesized brain abnormalities and biological dysfunctions while deemphasizing the centrality of the individual and their cultural and biopsychosocial context. Critics of the DSM and ICD have argued that disorders are arbitrary labels used to describe typical human experiences that are deemed abnormal. An example of this concept is that different countries have varied expectations and views of what is considered to be normal. A person who claims to talk to spirits might be considered schizophrenic in one culture while being deemed a holy person in another.

The DSM/ICD approach put the treatment utility of diagnosis and assessment on an indefinite hold, as if the ultimate purpose of such categorization—better outcomes—was an afterthought. The lack of treatment utility of the DSM/ICD was taken as a given instead of the shocking indication of failure that it is.

In response to all of these criticisms, the National Institute of Mental Health (NIMH) established the Research Domain Criteria (RDoC) framework, which aims to classify mental disorders based on dimensions of observable behavior and neurobiological measures (Insel et al., 2010). The RDoC framework proposed that underlying psychobiological abnormalities lead to observable patterns that overlap in various psychopathologies. Furthermore, the initiative used different levels of analyses—including molecular, brain circuit, symptom level, and behavioral—to define constructs that are proposed to be core symptoms of mental disorders.

Although RDoC put the focus on underlying processes, in its implementation it was almost entirely focused on biological processes, and it equated psychiatric problems with brain disorders (Hofmann & Hayes, 2019). Both the DSM/ICD and RDoC share the view that psychological distress is caused by a latent disease. Whereas in the DSM/ICD, the belief is that latent constructs are measured through clinical impressions and symptom reports, with RDoC, the view is that latent diseases can be measured with biological and behavioral tests. If the latent disease model itself is false, however, RDoC is too small of a step in the process direction. The lack of evidence for the latent disease model itself needs to be faced in order for practitioners to shift to a central focus on *processes of change*: the mechanisms that lead an individual to change, that are relevant for the individual in context, that provide increased treatment utility and intervention guidance, and that simplify human complexity.

Meanwhile, after the RDoC framework was established, practitioners, government entities, and the public in many parts of the world remained unconvinced about the value of evidence-based psychological care. Protocols were at times difficult to deploy, and the lack of known components and processes of change made them difficult to fit to individuals and their complexity. Most clients given psychosocial treatment did not receive evidence-based care.

WHAT DO CLINICIANS AND CLIENTS WANT FROM SCIENCE?

Virtually every clinician has encountered a person like Bill. And just like Sara, we can believe we made a difference in the client's life while still barely scratching the surface. Bill and Sara both may be drawn in by the focus on "depression" as something Bill "has" and miss the rich and important details of a man walking through a breakup that triggered deep-seated feelings of loneliness and inadequacy.

People are not diagnostic categories; they are suffering humans, each with their own story, history, and goals. Bill does not "have" depression. He feels depressed (and lonely, and disconnected) because of idiographic biopsychosocial factors, which also include his personal history, his past experience, and his maladaptive ways of coping with adversity.

Bill has his own story that brought him to the point of therapy. Individual human lives are contextual and longitudinal, as are the change processes that alter these life trajectories. Practitioners do not need to fit a set of pseudo-biomedical categories or labels for people's suffering to the person. Instead, they need coherent and broadly applicable models of the processes of change that need to occur—psychologically, biophysiologically, and socioculturally—so as to create desired long-term positive outcomes for the people they serve. Because processes of change are known to be functionally important pathways, a focus on treatment utility can be the *first* step in categorization, not the hoped-for step that never arrives. After all, increasing the likelihood of a truly good outcome is what clinicians and clients alike want from intervention science.

The most popular methodological and analytic tools in use in intervention science are not fully up to that task, even when they are turned in the direction of change processes. When we start fresh, however, we see new ways to frame human difficulties using other available methodological and analytic tools. We see new ways to make progress.

Processes of change represent proximal features of a clinical case over time that reliably predict long-term outcomes. Their proximal nature is important. For example, we know that changes in the way that clients talk about their thoughts and difficulties during early psychotherapy sessions can mediate follow-up outcomes, thus providing an early marker of real progress for practitioners to track in session. Unlike in other areas of expertise, clinicians don't get more competent with more experience, because they don't get immediate feedback on their practice. A process-based focus, however, may provide practitioners with the kind of immediate and functionally useful feedback necessary for experience to lead to expertise.

We define therapeutic processes of change as theory-based, dynamic, progressive, contextually bound, modifiable, and multilevel changes or mechanisms that occur in predictable, empirically established sequences and that can be used to produce desirable outcomes (note that this is a small refinement of Hofmann & Hayes, 2019, p. 38):

- **theory-based,** because we associate them with a clear scientific statement of relations among events that lead to testable predictions and methods of influence;

- **dynamic,** because they may involve feedback loops and nonlinear changes;

- **progressive,** because we may need to arrange them in particular sequences to reach the treatment goal;

- **contextually bound and modifiable,** because they directly suggest practical changes or treatment kernels within the reach of practitioners; and

- **multilevel,** because some processes supersede or are nested within others.

Finally, "it should be noted that the term *therapeutic process* is sometimes used in the literature to refer broadly to the patient-therapist relationship that includes so-called common factors, such as the therapeutic alliance and other factors of the therapeutic relationship. The term therapeutic process, as we use it, can include this more traditional use of the term as long as such processes are based on a clearly defined and testable theory, and meet the empirical standards we are suggesting. It is not, however, synonymous with that traditional use" (Hofmann & Hayes, 2019, p. 38). We will come back to this definition again in chapter 2 when we explain these different parts of the definition in more detail.

In the current paradigm of the medical model, evidence-based therapists either need to restrict their practice to specific syndromes or to acquire expertise in a wide variety of protocols for a variety of syndromes. This is untenable, impractical, and unreasonable and rests on invalid assumptions. The field has struggled to reach widespread resolution over many such issues, and the protocols-for-syndromes approach has failed to resolve them. It is our argument (Hofmann & Hayes, 2019) that intervention science needs to embrace and build on evidence-based processes of change linked to evidence-based procedures. It is time to move forward.

THE PROCESS-BASED ADVANTAGE

Each treatment approach carries with it its own assessment methods, terminology, and techniques that need to be tailored to the individual as necessary. The process-based vision is one of coherent sets of change processes that can be applied to a wide array of problem domains in an individually tailored manner—presenting practitioners with a less daunting training task of using change processes to fit treatment kernels to client needs. There is no need in this approach for a priori commitments to "schools" or "therapeutic orientation" or protocols. There are legitimate philosophical differences that need to be addressed, and models of change processes are needed to simplify and organize available evidence. But broad treatment schools, differences in orientation, and "brand name" interventions take a back seat to the individual needs of clients.

A process-oriented system can help diminish fruitless debates over levels of analysis (e.g., it's the brain; no, it's the therapeutic relationship) or preferred dimensions of psychological development (e.g., it's cognitive; no, it's behavioral) that are there even before the specific needs of a specific person are considered. Therapists and researchers would instead shift their focus to the most important biopsychosocial processes for a given client, given their goals and current circumstances, and to identifying the methods that best move them toward those goals with greater freedom to consider processes and methods across traditions and approaches (Hayes & Hofmann, 2018; Hofmann & Hayes, 2019).

Intervention guidance needs to be scientifically coherent, and it needs to have treatment utility that fits the needs of the individual (Hayes et al., 2019). Our argument for a process-based approach is that it will allow evidenced-based therapy to move beyond the pitfalls of protocols for syndromes that have slowed scientific and clinical progress and have made the notion of evidence-based therapy unpalatable to many. By targeting individual client needs and maintaining a focus on change processes, programs of intervention research can be developed that more fully integrate approaches focused on the individual (idiographic) and what we share with others (nomothetic).

This issue is not one of numerosity—it is one of level of analysis. Intensive, frequent assessment linked to dynamic network analyses (which we will describe in chapter 2) can be embedded in randomized controlled intervention trials. This allows a program of research to emerge that is sensitive to the individual as nomothetic questions are examined, without violating logical and statistical assumptions. The goal is to derive a theory-guided and testable model of the processes that are involved in treatment. Many of the procedures needed to target these processes are already known; they only need to be put together in a way to fit the individual (Hayes & Hofmann, 2018).

Such a vision of evidence-based therapy alters Gordon Paul's classic "clinical question" for evidence-based therapy, which drove the earliest days of behavior therapy. Instead of asking, "What treatment, by whom, is most effective for this individual with that specific problem, under which set of circumstances, and how does it come about?" (Paul, 1969; p. 44), a modern process-based approach asks, "What core biopsychosocial processes should be targeted with this client given this goal in this situation, and how can they most efficiently and effectively be changed?" (Hofmann & Hayes, 2019).

This change in the underlying question shifts attention away from identifying effective treatment packages for problem types to deploying effective treatment elements based on systems of therapeutic change processes. For example, instead of finding the best treatment for depression, the focus shifts to finding the best way to improve mood, reduce loneliness, and promote more meaningful and intimate relationships in a client who developed rigidity and patterns of emotional avoidance following the breakup of a relationship. That simple change might give Bill a vastly broader therapy experience and give Sara a richer set of evidence-based tools needed to address Bill's situation.

Our name for evidence-based therapy done in the pursuit of a process-based vision is *process-based therapy,* or *PBT.* PBT is not a new therapy—it is a new model of evidence-based therapy. The goal of PBT is to move toward understanding and targeting the processes of change in a given individual and to move away from nomothetic, group-based analyses that tend to miss important individual processes that may be vital for effective and efficient treatment. PBT emphasizes the importance of function over content and is based on identifying and testing key change processes that build upon each other in order to best treat the individual in a particular context at a particular point in time. As such, treatment is tailored to one's specific issues, in the present moment, while recognizing that effective treatments need not be limited to any one particular therapy orientation (e.g., behavioral or psychodynamic) or treatment strategy, but rather on the specific, measurable change processes that can solve individual problems and promote well-being.

CREATING A NEW FRAMEWORK

The field has tried a biomedical approach, pursuing a latent disease model, for half a century. This approach has been unsuccessful. We believe that enough is enough. The individual who is suffering cannot be reduced to a gene system, brain disorder, or neurotransmitter imbalance. For decades the development of evidence-based therapy has been based on experimental tests of protocols designed to impact psychiatric syndromes. As this paradigm weakens, a more process-based therapy approach is rising in its place, focused on how to best target and change core biopsychosocial processes in specific situations for given clients with given goals. This is an inherently more idiographic question than has normally been at issue in evidence-based therapy. In this book, we will outline methods of assessment and analysis that can integrate idiographic data and lead to nomothetic generalizations in a process-based era.

Questioning assumptions in science is disruptive. Within a defined area of study, a priori analytic assumptions provide the scaffolding for which questions are asked, which methods are used, and which data are deemed relevant. Professionals often view questions, methods, and analytic units simply as the required tools of good science—not reflections of assumptions—and as a result can experience a sense of disorientation when times of upheaval arrive and assumptions are pointed out and critically examined.

Shifting to a PBT framework requires reframing our questions in the field of clinical psychology from "What treatments work?" to "How do treatments work?" The aim of PBT is to best understand which core biopsychological processes to target in an individual given their specific goals and stage of intervention, and how to best do so, using functional analysis, complex network approaches, and identification of core change processes developed from evidence-based treatments (Hayes & Hofmann, 2018). The PBT approach involves identifying and addressing core change processes with a focus on the client's concerns.

Intervention involves using testable hypotheses to build upon the client's individual strengths and target problem areas in accordance with their goals. Syndromal classification treats individuals as belonging to a homogenous group, with the rationale that these individuals share the same underlying latent disease, even though decades of research have shown that even individuals with similar problems often experience different life challenges and trajectories. The syndromal approach has been given billions of dollars and decades of time to succeed. And still, it has not. It's time to change, even without financial support from Big Pharma and mainstream funding agencies.

Focusing on processes of change raises fundamental practical, methodological, and statistical issues that become more obvious once a standard diagnostic approach is abandoned. The "homogeneous populations" promised by DSM/ICD diagnostic categories were never achieved, but they delayed acknowledgment that without homogeneity it is mathematically impossible to generalize from analyses of groups to the individual (Gates & Molenaar, 2012). The field of clinical and psychological research is poised to apply person-specific statistical and treatment approaches—although more challenging—to further our knowledge of psychopathology and cognitive behavioral interventions. A process-based approach allows for this emphasis on the individual and their context and symptoms.

A FUNCTIONAL ANALYSIS TO TARGET PROCESSES OF CHANGE

PBT focuses on functionally important processes of change, ensuring treatment utility. Therefore, its goals, such as considering context and the utility of particular behaviors, are similar to those of classical functional analysis. However, PBT is broader in the range of processes considered and tailored toward clinician use. We stifle ourselves when we limit the application of evidence-based treatments to specific diagnoses, pigeon-holing ourselves into treating a specific group or applying a "name brand" method of intervention. Although diagnostically specific evidence-based treatments are typically based on well-established, effective methods, imagine how much more precise these treatments could be if they were tailored to the individual or their needs? Learning how to do that is the purpose of this book.

Functional analysis was originally used within behavioral therapy to describe the control of behavior by principles such as contingencies of reinforcement. It can be thought of as the identification and modification of relevant, impactful, and controllable processes that relate to an individual's specific behaviors. These relations can vary in strength depending on the amount of influence that variables have over one another.

Although many researchers have noted the importance of functional work, functional analysis has not been utilized to a high degree outside of traditional behavior analysis, where a focus on direct contingencies is still dominant. PBT is reemphasizing functional analysis, and we have recently (Hayes et al., 2019) described how to link the model we will present in this book to a new kind of *process-based functional analysis*, which we will cover in chapter 3. That, in turn, will be the vehicle for tailoring evidence-based procedures to relevant evidence-based processes.

To apply process-based functional analysis, therapeutic procedures and processes must be differentiated from one another. *Therapeutic procedures* are techniques that a therapist uses to reach a client's treatment goals (Hayes & Hofmann, 2018). *Therapeutic processes*, on the other hand, can be described as the underlying sequences of biopsychosocial changes that lead to the client's attaining their treatment goals (Hayes & Hofmann, 2018). How to apply this distinction will be addressed in detail as the book unfolds.

As clinicians, we monitor the function and circumstances of our clients' thoughts, emotions, attentional changes, sense of self, motivation, and behaviors in addition to increasing awareness of the biophysiological and sociocultural domains relevant to our clients' goals. By examining these areas in terms of processes of change and relating data to intervention decisions, we can have concrete tools to apply an evidence-based functional analytic framework to identify and target processes of change that help clients achieve their goals.

A META-MODEL OF TREATMENT TARGETS

Clinicians differ in their therapeutic orientations, their preconceptions, and even their favorite therapeutic strategies. As a result, the same client could encounter a variety of therapists with different approaches. PBT does not restrict variation in these clinical approaches. In fact, PBT encourages clinicians to consider evidence-based processes that arose outside their own therapeutic approach and to use those that work best for their client.

Therefore, PBT needs to be based on a view of intervention that accommodates any evidence-based change processes, regardless of the specific therapeutic orientation. For this, we need a comprehensive, internally coherent, and functional system to organize PBT processes. The theoretical foundations of this meta-model are grounded in evolutionary principles that help us understand the development of complex systems in the life sciences. Our *Extended Evolutionary Meta-Model* (EEMM) provides consilience and a common language for such a system (Hayes, Hofmann, & Wilson, in press). As we will discuss, the EEMM applies the evolutionary concepts of context-appropriate variation, selection, and retention to key biopsychosocial dimensions and levels related to human suffering, problems, and positive functioning. That is the essence of PBT and the applied purpose of this skills training manual. Let the journey begin.

Action Step 1.1   Identify a Problem

In each chapter we will periodically stop and ask you to apply what we are talking about in short "action step" exercises. These exercises are also available to download from the website for this book, http://www.newharbinger.com/47551. (See the very back of this book for more details.) In some of these we will ask you to explore these ideas by applying them to your own life. We do that for two reasons. One is because you know the details of your life and can bring that rich history to the task. The other is that you can get more of an intuitive or felt sense of how these perspectives actually land when you try to apply them to yourself. For many of these exercises, we will provide an example of a response. So please keep a notebook or digital device handy as you read the book, and let's dive in to our first action step.

Please pick one or two problem areas in your life that, if you were to seek psychological help, might be areas you would pick to work on. They may have a long or short history—the only requirement is that they are present today. Your task is simply to write a paragraph describing each problem area, much as you might in an initial consultation with a provider. Supply whatever details you consider meaningful.

We are suggesting you consider "one or two" problem areas because from the next chapter on we will refer back to whatever problem area you choose, and it may take some thought to narrow your focus to one that best fits the purposes of these action step exercises and that feels sufficiently important. If you know now that a particular one is best, just go with that.

Next, based only on what you know from previous training, try to label what you wrote using only DSM/ICD diagnoses. Feel free to use "not otherwise specified" or adjustment disorder. If you feel you must use multiple diagnoses, you may.

Finally, write a short paragraph about what feelings and thoughts you have when you think about the DSM/ICD label. Where does your mind go? How do you react when you look at the problem areas through the lens of the DSM/ICD?

Below is an example of how someone might complete this exercise. We will follow this same person throughout our action step examples.

Example

Problem Area: I get anxious and insecure when talking to others, especially with people I do not know, people I consider attractive, or people in higher positions of power. I notice I get stuck in my head, worry about what they think of me, worry that they might not like me. As a result, I retreat more and more inside my head. I worry about saying something stupid and embarrassing myself. I deal with these fears by either overcompensating and trying to be the most fun and interesting person in the room or by retreating, excusing myself from the situation and going home. These fears have been with me as long as I can remember.

DSM/ICD Diagnosis: Social anxiety disorder/social phobia

What Feelings and Thoughts Come Up for Me: The DSM label feels overly simplistic and threatening at the same time. It feels like all the complexity of my situation is compressed into a single label. And it feels like confirmation that there is something wrong with who I am. Something is broken inside of me, and I'm less of a person because of it. It also sounds like I need medication to fix my problem.

CHAPTER 2

The Network Approach

When we let go of the idea of trying to fit clients into DSM/ICD-shaped molds, we can move to a more useful and progressive approach. This new approach reflects the reality of the client much better because it is focused on what science can tell us about the client's struggles, and what needs to be done to meet their needs and accomplish their goals. We call it the process-based approach. In this chapter, we'll look at the first element of the process-based approach—the network model—which depicts the client's current situation, personal history, and every other process you might choose to target. This network model will form the basis of our work with the client. But before we can get there, let's first define the basic terms.

WHAT IS A PROCESS?

The word "process" comes from a Latin root meaning "going forward," as in a parade or a procession, and its modern definition—*a series of actions meant to accomplish some result*—has existed for 400 years. A process in PBT is a sequence of events that is known to influence a person's well-being. It can be a direct influence (for instance, regular exercise directly influences your well-being), or it can be an indirect influence (for instance, knowing someone who regularly works out can inspire you to exercise more, which in turn influences your well-being). At any given moment, a multitude of processes happen simultaneously within every person, interacting with other processes and affecting a person's well-being.

Not all processes have a positive influence. In fact, many processes have a negative effect on a person's well-being, such as avoiding feelings of anxiety or suppressing a traumatic memory. What's more, the same event can lead to maladaptive processes in some people and adaptive ones in others despite their superficial similarity. For instance, the early death of a parent could throw one person who is unable to face the grief into a cycle of social withdrawal, misery, and despair, while causing another person when facing grief to grow connected to loved ones and resilient when confronted by the stressors of life. It depends on the individual person, their context, and the specific processes in play.

There is a virtually unlimited number of biopsychosocial processes active within every person, which is why we want to limit ourselves to the ones that are relevant to clinical interventions. The general term "processes of change" can apply to both maladaptive and adaptive processes. Maladaptive processes are especially therapeutically relevant in terms of diagnosis, functional analysis, and negative targets of intervention, while adaptive processes provide positive targets to be strengthened. When processes of change are relevant to reaching therapeutic goals, they are *therapeutic processes*. They come in many shapes and forms, yet all of the most useful therapeutic processes exhibit the same five qualities. As a reminder, therapeutic processes are theory-based, dynamic, progressive, contextually bound, and part of a multilevel system. We briefly defined these five qualities in the last chapter; here, let's unpack their meanings further.

Theory-based: A therapeutic process is associated with a clear statement of relations among events that lead to testable predictions. For example, suppose a particular theory emphasized how thoughts of possible humiliation lead to strong emotions in social situations that then make social functioning difficult. A process concept like that might lead you to perk up when a client who is socially avoidant says, "I am worried that people will laugh at me." It would cause you to look carefully for signs of increased anxiety that inhibit social behavior. A process is not a single event—it is a conceptually predicted relationship between one event (e.g., thinking, *People will laugh at me*) and other events (feeling anxiety and being less functional socially).

Dynamic: A therapeutic process involves feedback loops and nonlinear changes. For example, suppose a person has the thought *I'm worthless* and believes it. That combination might lead them to forego basic hygienic routines, such as bathing. The social response of others (e.g., a wrinkled-up nose or snide comments) in turn can encourage them to believe the thought that they are worthless even more. Thus, believing the thought *I'm worthless,* lack of hygiene, and a social expression of disgust from others are now in a self-reinforcing feedback loop, where each event strengthens the others in a self-amplifying process.

Progressive: A therapeutic process may need to be arranged in particular sequence to reach the treatment goal. For instance, it may not be enough to merely identify that a client's craving for cocaine leads to drug consumption. If we want treatment to be successful, we also need to uncover the values violations that have occurred as a result of the addiction in order for the client to have enough motivation to do anything different with the craving. The right sequence of processes helps you reach the treatment goal.

Contextual: A therapeutic process needs to be contextually bound and modifiable so that it is within your reach to directly suggest practical changes or treatment kernels. For instance, no amount of therapy will be able to undo the sexual abuse a client has experienced in their life. However, the history of sexual abuse may affect many aspects of the client's life in the here and now, which is where you can intervene, such as the conditions under which distrust of others leads to excessive testing of intimate partners in an effort to feel safer. A "history of sexual abuse" is itself not contextually bound or modifiable, but because it does its damage in part due to processes of change that occur in particular situations (trying to modify a feeling produced by that history in the context of intimate relationships), the key therapeutic processes are within reach of your interventions.

Multilevel: A therapeutic process may supersede other processes or may be nested within another process. For instance, a lack of concentration may lead to a client's outbursts of crying because of a sense of shame…but that process may be nested within unhealthy entanglement with thoughts of blame over the death of a partner. By focusing on the process of grief linked to self-blame, other processes may become obsolete or be put in a new, larger perspective.

These are the five qualities of therapeutic processes, and it's worth keeping these qualities in mind when we want to make sense of a client's situation. By focusing on therapeutic change processes that are in line with these five qualities, we can bring together clinical practitioners from many different theoretical backgrounds. Oftentimes, there are parallel concepts in different schools of clinical psychology. But while it's often difficult to come to an agreement on overall models, common interest in processes of change is far easier to establish. And if we see processes that exemplify the qualities mentioned above, we can consider them as building blocks for an alternative approach to the DSM/ICD.

In process-based therapy, we use change processes to go beyond the traditional DSM/ICD model and create an approach that has known treatment utility—because it focuses on processes that are already known to be functionally important in leading to long-term positive or negative outcomes. And in order to take this step, we need to ensure that the concepts we use to describe and explain therapeutic processes have the following three qualities:

Precision: A therapeutic process needs precision so that it is clear when a particular change process can be said to apply and when it cannot. For instance, a concept like "avoiding" is less precise than a concept such as "avoiding intense feelings." By requiring change processes to be precise, we eliminate general heuristics and loose metaphors as processes of change.

Scope: A therapeutic process needs scope so that it applies to a range of phenomena. For instance, a process that focuses on "verbal quarrels with intimate friends" has less scope than a process such as "fostering emotional distance through quarrels, refusals, and withdrawal." By requiring change processes to have scope, we eliminate those that are merely restated versions of specific psychological episodes, and we encourage those that broadly apply to a client's psychosocial world. It is simply not useful—neither scientifically nor practically—to focus on processes that apply only to narrow areas.

Depth: Clinical psychology is embedded in a broad pool of scientific knowledge drawn from neuroscience, physiology, genetics, social processes, and many other disciplines. As such, a therapeutic process needs depth so that evidence is consistent with well-established scientific findings at different levels of analysis. For instance, if an emotional process concept contradicts data from the neurobiology of emotion, something is deeply wrong. If there is such a contradiction in the fabric of science, the description of the change process is not yet adequate.

At any given moment, there are a multitude of different processes of change interacting simultaneously within a client. These processes are linked to the person's feelings, thoughts, behaviors, sense of self, and even their biological, social, and cultural experiences. If we want to do justice to the client and depict their situation with all its complexity in a structured, practical way, we need a reliable, simple approach to organize client information and features into a process-based account. We believe that challenge can be met by taking a network approach.

NETWORK THINKING

Network models are often used to make sense of dynamic and interconnected systems. For example, climate scientists rely on network models to make sense of changes in temperature and weather across the globe. Stock market experts apply network models to track and predict the rise and fall of individual shares. And we too will use network models to bring clarity to a client's history, current situation, and likely treatment response.

A network is made up of single parts that link together and influence one another. In PBT, we create network models using squares and arrows, whereby two squares link to each other by an arrow. The squares represent the events of a person's life that are related to functioning. And the arrows between these squares represent the relation between these events and their direction of influence.

Simple Relation

To get a basic idea of how the network model works, take a look at figure 2.1.

In this case a historical fact ("History of being bullied") reinforces the event "Low self-esteem," as depicted by an arrow. By drawing multiple squares, each representing a different event, that are connected with multiple arrows, we can create a model of a client's situation.

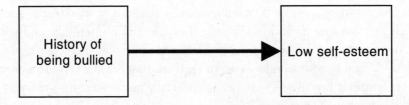

Figure 2.1 Simple relation

Processes are sequences, and in the example above the arrow is clearly a process; the history of bullying led to an internalization—low self-esteem. In general terms, being treated badly led to believing *I'm bad*. But the low self-esteem can also be a process if it then changes how other events are handled—for example, how criticism from others is perceived.

The network approach is not only useful to capture relevant processes in a client's life. We can also use this model to make meaningful statements about how these individual processes interact and reinforce one another. As we draw different relations between the individual squares, we are explicating possible process relations. In time, you'll find a client's network expand from a simple relation to multiple squares with complex relations.

Complex Relations

Events can be linked to each other in many different ways. You have already seen the first example, where one event influences a second event. It does not get easier than this. Now suppose two events are in a feedback loop, where they influence and reinforce each other. For example, a person with a fear of dogs might avoid dogs at all costs, but that very act of avoidance may also maintain and reinforce their fear. The first event reinforces a second event, which in turn reinforces the first, repeating the cycle. Take a look at figure 2.2 to see what this relation would look like in the network approach.

Whenever two squares make a feedback loop, we have a process that can maintain itself or build on itself, either positively or negatively. For example, when a person has experienced a panic attack, they may start to avoid situations in which the panic attack has been triggered, hoping to avert possible future panic attacks. As a result, they become more vigilant, cautious, and agitated about their anxiety, which increases the odds of triggering yet another panic attack, making them retreat even more. And while their area of comfort is getting smaller and smaller, their panic attacks increase in size and frequency. In such a case, a "Panic attack" and "Avoidance of anxiety-provoking situations" are in a constant feedback loop, reinforcing and building on each other. And once they are in a feedback loop, they tend to select and maintain their elements, becoming less sensitive to context and more resistant to change. The process term "experiential avoidance" describes such a network.

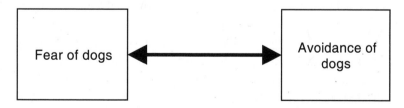

Figure 2.2 Feedback loop

In most cases, more than just two events interact with each other. So let's add one more square to our model, making room for an additional event, and see how it influences the network. Take a look at figure 2.3.

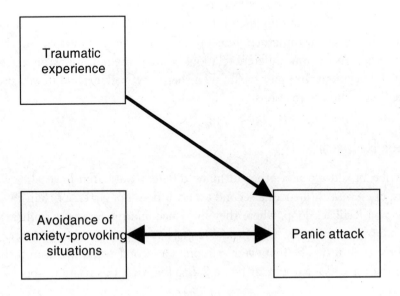

Figure 2.3 Three-way relation

In this case, the process "Panic attack" is in a direct feedback loop with "Avoidance of anxiety-provoking situations." Note that "Avoidance of anxiety-provoking situations" is itself a process relation—and we could have drawn it as a series of smaller pieces, such as "situation," "anxiety," and "avoidance"—but networks rapidly become unreadable if we break them down into tiny pieces, so there is no rule against putting processes in boxes. Additionally, we included in the model the role of a "Traumatic experience" that provoked the initial panic attack in the first place.

Now we have three interlinked squares in our model, but we are not done yet. Suppose the process "Traumatic experience" has a much stronger influence on the process "Panic attack" than the process "Avoidance of anxiety-provoking situations" does. We can depict the strength of a relation by adjusting the size of the arrowhead accordingly.

In figure 2.4, the arrow leading from "Traumatic experience" now has a much bigger arrowhead, indicating that "Traumatic experience" has a much stronger influence on the event "Panic attack" than "Avoidance of anxiety-provoking situations" does.

We already talked about feedback loops occurring between two events, leading to a self-reinforcing loop (as in figure 2.2). In reality, it's just as common to find feedback loops between three or more events.

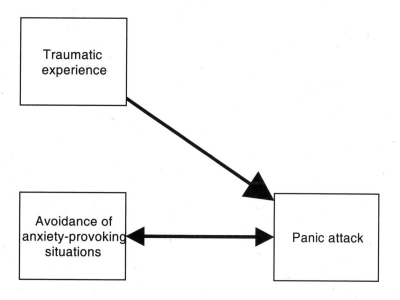

Figure 2.4 Stronger influence

We already talked about feedback loops occurring between two events, leading to a self-reinforcing loop (as in figure 2.2). In reality, it's just as common to find feedback loops between three or more events. Let's take a look at figure 2.5.

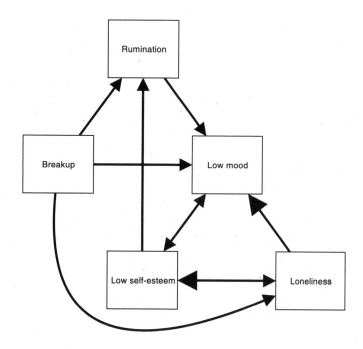

Figure 2.5 Subnetwork

There is a lot going on in this network model, so let's go through it bit by bit. This client has recently gone through a breakup from her boyfriend, which led her to frequently ruminate about the past. The event "Breakup" has a direct impact on lowering the client's overall mood as well as leading her to ruminate about the past (which in turn lowers the client's mood further). Those three squares are connected by single-headed arrows, suggesting that rumination is part of a functionally important pathway that bridges the impact of the breakup on low mood. Simple unidirectional networks like this are commonly modeled in studies of the "mediation" of treatment outcomes in randomized controlled trials.

But then the overall network gets more complicated, and self-amplifying loops begin to appear. As a consequence of the breakup, the client is struggling with loneliness, which in turn feeds low self-esteem *and* is reinforced by the low self-esteem itself. The loneliness, in turn, contributes to the client's low mood. And the low self-esteem, in turn, leads the client to ruminate more often, which also fosters low mood.

We call these self-reinforcing patterns *subnetworks*: smaller networks within the larger network that are autonomous to a degree because of feedback loops sustained in the smaller network. A bidirectional relation between two events is the simplest subnetwork, but we tend to reserve the term "subnetwork" for small networks containing three or more events.

In this client's case, we can identify two primary subnetworks. The first one is between the nodes "Low self-esteem," "Loneliness," and "Low mood," which bring together affective, cognitive, and self-related aspects in a single subsystem. The client feels lonely, which reinforces her feelings of low mood, which in turn lowers her concept of herself (low self-esteem). Low self-esteem, in turn, reinforces her feelings of loneliness, repeating the cycle.

There is also a second subnetwork, between the processes "Low self-esteem," "Rumination," and "Low mood." This brings together issues of self, cognition, and affect into a single interlocked and self-sustaining system. The client's low self-esteem leads her to ruminate about the past, which in turn lowers her mood, which—yet again—contributes to her low self-esteem. Again, it's a self-reinforcing cycle, where three or more psychological events influence and reinforce each other in a system of change processes.

Note that "Low self-esteem" and "Low mood" are involved in both subnetworks, giving both a key role in the maintenance of a client's problems. Additionally, the process "Loneliness" has a strong direct influence on "Low self-esteem" and "Low mood" (as shown by the larger arrowheads), giving it a key role as well. If you want to disrupt the client's network, targeting reactions to loneliness, low mood, or low self-esteem could thus all be sensible ways to do so. This idea—that the processes of change involved in multiple subnetworks are often especially good ones to target in therapy—is a key feature of process-based diagnosis.

These are the most important relations you need to know to get started working with the network model. The network should be as complex as necessary and as simple as possible. In other words, we need to add as many events and relations to the model as necessary to identify the key processes of change, yet simultaneously as few as possible to keep the model clear, simple, and practical. We will give some preliminary guidance about how you can do that in this chapter and will expand these ideas in the next chapter on the Extended Evolutionary Meta-Model, or EEMM (pronounced "eem" as in "team").

Depending on the treatment goal, it may be useful to exclude a certain number of otherwise important events in the client's life. For instance, an absent father figure may have no influence on a person's habit of drug abuse and should thus be excluded from a network model that is aimed at helping this person overcome processes that foster drug addiction. Pick only those events that have a relevant direct or indirect influence on your therapeutic goal in the form of empirically established and changeable processes of change.

Once you have developed a client's network model, you can use it to make meaningful statements about what led to a problem, which factors maintain it, how the problem might progress, and where you might effectively intervene to guide the client toward a meaningful change. In order to know which processes are the most important in any given network model—in other words, which processes maintain the network and which are most susceptible to change—you need to know how to analyze the network model you have constructed.

ANALYZING A NETWORK MODEL

The network model can help you gain important insights about the client. Merely by looking at the model, you can conclude which life events are the most relevant, how events engage other events, how events form a process that maintains the client's problems, how these processes relate to one another, how strong their respective influence is, and what their larger role is within the network. As a rule of thumb, an event becomes more important to the network when it has a strong influence on another event or when it influences multiple other processes within the network. Take a look at figure 2.6.

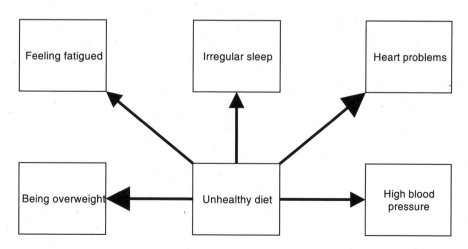

Figure 2.6 One event influences many

In this case, an "Unhealthy diet" affects a multitude of other events, including "Being over-weight," "Feeling fatigued," "Irregular sleep," "Heart problems," and "High blood pressure." For this client, an "Unhealthy diet" is thus highly important to the larger network and therefore offers an excellent starting point for clinical intervention once the clinician and client understand the processes that are sustaining, and might alter, this unhealthy eating.

There is also the reverse case, where one event is influenced by a multitude of other adjacent events. Take a look at figure 2.7.

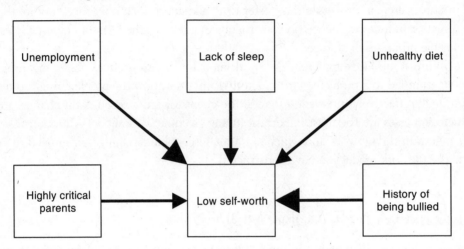

Figure 2.7 Many events influence one

In this case, "Low self-worth" is reinforced by such events as "Highly critical parents," "Unemployment," "Lack of sleep," "Unhealthy diet," and "History of being bullied." Many things influence a person's self-worth. In this case, past and present social and cultural factors (being bullied, critical parents, and unemployment) and lifestyle factors (unhealthy diet and lack sleep) seem most relevant. There might be other factors that have not been explored yet. Perhaps certain behaviors and thoughts, for example, also contribute to this person's self-worth. As we will describe later, the EEMM will give us a guide to systematically explore other possible factors.

Although low self-worth plays an important role in the network, the very fact that it is supported by so many other features of the network suggests that it might not be a good starting point for clinical intervention. Low self-worth may be more resilient to change because it is reinforced by multiple other events, some of which (e.g., the history of being bullied; critical parents) may be either impossible or difficult to change. As a result, it may be more useful to change the processes that feed into low-self-worth first. For example, this client may have a rigid cognitive style that readily leads to strong self-criticism whenever negative events occur, such as the five shown in this network.

A network might be resistant to change until it reaches a tipping point in a specific process. An important sign of an impending tipping point is a critical speeding up or slowing down in the network model. For example, when a person needs less time to recover from a stressor, it might indicate a tipping point from maladaptation to health. In contrast, when a person needs more time to recover, it can indicate a tipping point from health to dysfunction. Whenever you witness a change of pace from one state of a network to another, it is wise to pay attention.

By looking at a network model in this manner, you can draw meaningful conclusions about the effect different events have on one another and on the network at large, especially once it is backed up by longitudinal measurements, as we will discuss later in the book. You can see which events lead to a problem, which processes maintain that relationship, and how a problem might progress in the future, depending on which processes reinforce the problem.

The network models of real-life people are often more complex than the ones we have shown in the examples. There are often far more events and processes involved, interacting and relating to each other in more complex ways. But again, do not worry about it getting too complicated, as we will get there step by step. So let's apply the network approach to an actual person and see what it looks like in practice.

APPLYING A NETWORK APPROACH

Throughout this book, we will follow different clients as we walk through the principles and practice of process-based therapy. These individuals are a product of fiction, and any resemblance to any real-life person is not intended and entirely coincidental. Nonetheless, they have been inspired by our therapeutic experience, and we have written their cases in a way to resemble real-life clients you might encounter in your therapeutic practice. This being said, let's meet our first client and see what we learn about her during our first conversation.

Andrea is a sixty-one-year-old woman who frequently worries about the well-being of her loved ones. She calls her thirty-year-old daughter at least once a day and anxiously inquires about her well-being; about her granddaughter's childcare, diet, seat belt use, and ability to make friends (and whether the parents of her friends have been "vetted"); about her daughter's driving speed; about the use of pool floatation devices; and about a thousand other similar concerns. Andrea is convinced she is likely to die soon, so she frequently visits the doctor's office, demanding expensive medical tests. And when the results come back negative, she either questions the physician's competence and demands a second test or feels reassured but only for a few hours or days before she begins worrying again. She also asks her current husband for reassurance several times a day, in matters such as his health, where he is, whether he thinks she is looking flushed, whether a skin bump on her back might be cancer, and similar matters. Her husband is supportive but struggles to understand where these anxious requests are coming from.

In our first conversation with Andrea, we already learned a great deal about her difficulties and how they are affecting the life of her loved ones and those around her. If we want to represent her case in a network model, we first need to identify the important life events. A common theme in her life is the frequent worry about her own health and the well-being of her loved ones. And whenever she worries, she asks her loved ones—either her daughter or her husband—for reassurance. This brings her initial relief, until she worries again and repeats the cycle. Additionally, she deals with her worry by taking medical tests, which sometimes brings her temporary relief (until she begins worrying again), and other times leads her to doubt the test results (when they come back negative), leading her to retake the medical tests. If we put these insights into a network, it might look similar to figure 2.8.

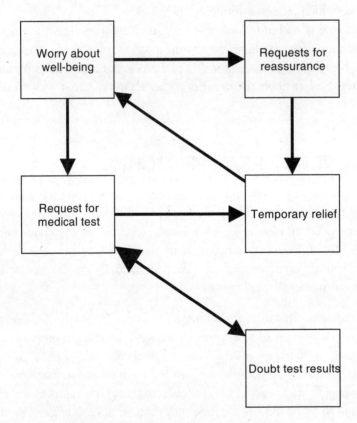

Figure 2.8 Andrea's network model

Take a minute to look at the individual events as well as their interconnected relations in figure 2.8. As you can see, the upper four events are in two interconnected feedback loops, where "Worry about well-being" eventually leads to "Temporary relief"—either by requesting reassurance from her loved ones or by taking more medical tests. The temporary relief, however, eventually leads back to worrying in a never-ending cycle.

Both of these loops are instances of the same processes of change: forms of reassurance diminishing worry but also feeding the central role of worry, thus strengthening the loop. There are various names for loops of this kind ("experiential avoidance" is one). Additionally, the events "Request for medical test" and "Doubt test results" are in a direct feedback loop, causing one another. Notice that the arrow that moves from "Doubt test results" to "Request for medical test" is much stronger than the other way around, because a medical test does not always lead to doubting the test results, but doubting the test results almost always leads to taking more medical tests.

This is what a network model can look like in practice. By conceptualizing a clinical case using such a model, we can view psychopathology as something that continually shifts and changes over time, emphasizing transition between states of pathology and health. It also enables us to draw direct relations between different features of a client's life rather than having to rely on the assumption that symptoms are expressions of underlying diseases. These individualized network models—tailormade to fit the client's individual situation—can then be used to inform treatment strategies by identifying those processes that are most important and most susceptible to change.

Action Step 2.1   Create a Network Model

Let's return to one of the problem areas in your own life. Draw a network of events that seem to characterize it. Focus more on what appears to be present now and less about where it might have come from based on events in the distant past. Use single- or double-headed arrows to describe what leads to what in your experience. Try to keep the network small, with six nodes or fewer. Keep in mind that you can always alter your network as you go along.

Next, write a short paragraph about what happens for you when you think this way. What feelings and thoughts come up for you? How do you react when you look at this problem through the lens of this network?

Following the example we used in Action Step 1.1, below we illustrate how that person might have completed this exercise.

Example

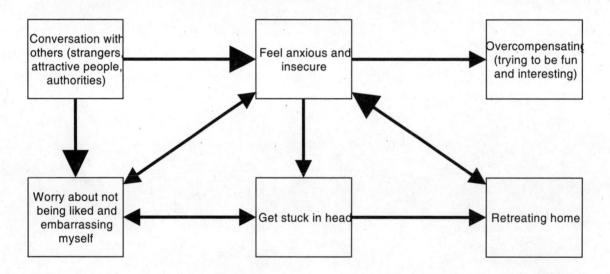

What Feelings and Thoughts Come Up for Me: I never thought about my problem in this way. The nodes help show a good overview of all the elements, and the arrows show how they influence one another. I never before stopped to think about how everything reinforces each other. Drawing this network helped me make more sense of my situation. My problem feels like something I can learn to get a better grip on.

CHAPTER 3

The Extended Evolutionary Meta-Model

Throughout the history of psychology, clinicians have found many different ways to talk about therapeutic change processes. Sigmund Freud and psychoanalysts talked about working through unconscious defense mechanisms and infantile sexual drives. Aaron T. Beck and followers of cognitive therapy focused on changes in automatic thoughts and core beliefs. Other scientists and therapists used completely different terminology to describe and categorize therapeutic change processes in countless other ways.

The many ways to talk about change processes is not only confusing to clients—it also complicates communication among clinicians, making it difficult for them to compare and translate change processes into therapy. If we wish to stop this needless complexity, study and practice psychotherapy effectively, and serve clients to the best of our abilities, we need to find a common language for talking about therapeutic change processes. That has long been recognized, but the task is difficult.

Past attempts have already been made to integrate information about change processes across a wide range of therapies. However, these attempts have been built on top of specific theoretical models, limiting the application for different schools of thought. In process-based therapy (PBT), we aim to give all processes from all streams of psychotherapy a fair chance to be considered, based on their proven usefulness for achieving a therapeutic goal rather than the adherence to specific psychological theories.

But therapeutic processes that are to be considered for PBT need to meet certain criteria. In the previous chapter, we talked about the five key qualities of therapeutic change processes, namely that they need to be theory-based, dynamic, progressive, contextually bound, and part of a multilevel system. Furthermore, these change processes need to have precision, scope, and depth. But how can we identify processes that fit these criteria and then fit them into a coherent system that all wings of clinical work can use? And how can we know which change processes are most useful and relevant for achieving a therapeutic goal? In order to answer these questions, we need to turn to every psychologist's best friend: the wonderful world of statistics.

MEDIATORS

The primary way researchers have studied therapeutic change processes is through *mediators* (i.e., the variables that change as a result of treatment and that produce the treatment outcome). In case it has been some time since your last statistics class, we'll give you a little refresher. In 1986 researchers Reuben Baron and David Kenny wrote one of the most highly cited articles in the entire field of science in which they defined a mediator as "the generative mechanism through which the focal independent variable is able to influence the dependent variable of interest" (Baron & Kenny, 1986, p. 1173).

For example, suppose we observe that some employees of a company tend to eat more fast food during the holiday session. In other words, holiday season (the independent variable) has an effect on eating fast food (the dependent variable). Upon taking a closer look, however, let's imagine that we notice that the holiday season leads to greater stress at work, which in turn leads to eating more fast food. In other words, work distress acts as a mediator: a functionally important pathway through which the independent variable ("holiday season") influences the dependent variable ("eating fast food"). As shown in figure 3.1, work distress is a functionally important pathway of change by which the holiday season leads to unhealthy eating.

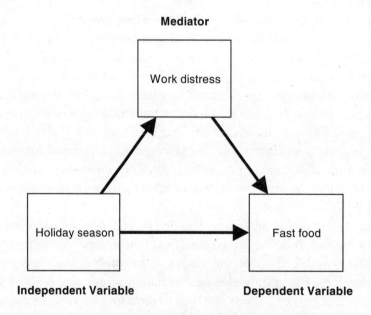

Figure 3.1 An example of mediation

Suppose when the influence of work distress is statistically removed, the holiday season no longer leads people to eat more fast food. This finding could suggest very practical ways of dealing with the issue. Perhaps we try adding more employees during the holiday season and thereby reducing the work stress of each employee. If fast food eating is then completely unrelated to the holiday season because work stress is eliminated, we would be able to speak statistically of "full mediation." If we erase the mediator ("work distress") by our intervention, and the effect of the independent variable ("holiday season") on the dependent variable ("eating fast food") completely disappears, then that label would apply. If, however, there is still an effect between the independent variable and the dependent variable even after accounting for the mediator, we could speak of "partial mediation." In this case, the holiday season still has some effect on eating more fast food, regardless of work distress, perhaps because some holidays make fast food more desirable (or for some other reason we don't know).

If we can reliably show a process acting as a mediator between a clinical intervention and an outcome, it can have therapeutic value. This is a big reason why we focused on mediational research in the first place. Syndromal diagnosis (as in the DSM and ICD) does not have known treatment utility. Mediators, on the other hand, have proven treatment utility and are by definition functionally important to clinical outcomes when they are changed by intervention.

As a method, mediation admittedly has some shortcomings. For one thing, it can handle only a very small number of variables. As additional variables are added, the statistical models become more complex, less powerful, and harder to interpret. For that reason, generally only one or two mediators are examined empirically at a time—but these "pauci-variate" models do not fit the real world, nor do they fit our models of change. No one believes that a single variable is responsible for most positive changes in life.

Perhaps even more importantly, mediation assumes that processes of change are related in a linear way to treatment and then to outcome (controlling for treatment). That is even less likely. Psychological change is rarely, if ever, a linear and unidirectional process—as outcomes change, processes also change.

When both of these issues are combined, mediation as it is studied now has notable limitations. Treatment change is a dynamic process that involves many variables often forming bidirectional and interrelated connections that form networks and subnetworks, such as positive and negative feedback loops (Hofmann, Curtiss, & Hayes, 2020). Psychological treatments involve many possible variables. When reviewing the CBT literature, we find that cognitive and behavioral strategies appear to be the change processes when treating anxiety and depression (Kazantzis et al., 2018). However, this literature is relatively small. We believe that the processes we take into consideration in a PBT approach need to begin with what the world's literature tells us about successful mediators of clinically important outcomes. In a large meta-analysis we are soon to publish of randomized clinical trials targeting psychological outcomes, statistically significant mediation has been found five or more times for forty different processes of change: experiential avoidance (or its flip side of acceptance) has been noted at least fifty-two times; self-efficacy has been found sixty-nine times; cognitive reappraisal, dysfunctional thoughts, or dysfunctional beliefs forty-seven times; mindfulness forty-one times; and so on (Hayes, Hofmann, Ciarrochi, et al., 2020). We will summarize a few key findings from that meta-analysis in chapter 8. We wanted to focus on process variables that regularly work as mediators because, even given the limitations of mediational analysis, we know that regularly identified mediators can comprise functionally important avenues of change under at least some conditions.

Change processes form complex sets of relationships, ultimately determining how change happens. PBT has developed a strategy for making sense of this complexity—an overarching framework to accommodate the complex nature of these processes.

MAKING SENSE OF PROCESSES

There is no point to using hundreds of therapeutic change processes to guide assessment and treatment. The list is simply too long to be practical. Instead, we must simplify and shorten the list by relying on both theory and evidence. We will use the term "model" to describe a conceptually integrated set of change processes that are used as a guide to select and deploy psychological interventions so as to achieve positive outcomes.

Such a model will have to meet a range of criteria. First, it will need to cover enough change processes over a sufficient range of problems to serve as a practical guide for psychological care. Second, the processes identified within the model will need to address a range of key elements of the human experience, such as motivation to change, sense of self, and affect. Ideally, the processes selected will focus not only on ameliorating problems but also on helping people prosper and thrive. Third, if models of change processes are to become the basis of an alternative to the DSM or ICD, then they must be few and they must be able to be compared empirically. Scores and scores of models are just as practically problematic as scores and scores of diagnoses. Fourth, the processes of change included in any given model must fit together in a coherent fashion, and evidence must show that the set is complete. Fifth, a model of change processes needs to be practical: it should lead to new forms of functional analysis that allow practitioners to select those treatment elements that produce better outcomes. Last, the model must be applicable across a broad range of clients from all walks of life and different cultural backgrounds.

Finally, the way we talk about different models must reflect consilience. One of the biggest benefits of the DSM/ICD is having a common communicating system, and it is worth trying to develop such a common set of concepts within process-based approaches. Among all available alternatives, only one overarching approach seems to be available that has the weight and breadth needed to meet all the previously mentioned criteria. This approach is the mother of all theories in the life sciences: the theory of evolution.

THE SIX KEY CONCEPTS IN EVOLUTION

In 1973, evolutionary biologist Theodosius Dobzhansky famously declared that "nothing in biology makes sense except in the light of evolution" (Dobzhansky, 1973). With this statement, he highlighted the fact that no biological process was born out of thin air but emerged over time based on changes and conditions described by evolutionary theory. Nowadays, it is undoubtedly accepted in the life sciences that any function of any life form has an evolutionary explanation.

This approach has not yet taken hold in the behavioral and cognitive sciences. Part of the problem is that evolutionary perspectives went through an era of "gene centrism" in the last century. Evolutionary biologist Richard Dawkins's influential book *The Selfish Gene* (Dawkins, 1976) is an example. It encouraged an evolutionary perspective cast largely in terms of genetic changes. However, the mapping of the human genome proved that this view is too narrow for our purposes in clinical psychology; enormous studies with several hundred thousand fully mapped human genomes showed that the vast majority of mental health issues are impacted by hundreds if not thousands of genes in incremental and extremely complex ways. Gene-centric thinking cannot account for behavior in a direct or simple way.

This does not mean genes do not matter. They do—but as part of entire networks of evolving dimensions, including epigenetic regulation of gene systems, neurobiological processes, environment, behavior, learning, development, symbolic events, culture, the gut biome, and so on. As science has shifted toward a modern multidimensional, multilevel "extended evolutionary account," it has become much easier to extend an evolutionary umbrella over process-based systems in the behavioral sciences.

There are six key concepts needed in an evolutionary approach, which can be expressed in the acronym VRSCDL (pronounced as the word "versatile"), which stands for **V**ariation and **R**etention of what is **S**elected in **C**ontext at the right **D**imension and **L**evel. In a well-rounded evolutionary account, these concepts are applied to any phenomenon using Niko Tinbergen's (1963) four central questions of function, history, development, and mechanism. Let's unpack what those key concepts mean in the context of clinical psychology.

Variation: Variation in evolution means that there are always slightly different forms available in any living system—different bodily forms, different sensitivities, different action. Initially variation is blind (i.e., random and entirely purposeless), but because variation is so central to the successful development of complex systems, variation itself evolves and becomes controlled by context, allowing for a broader range of alternatives when they might be most needed. In a sense, variation becomes "purposive." Even bacteria show these effects. If an essential amino acid is removed from a food source, almost immediately bacteria will start mutating, as if to "find another way." Extinction effects are a good and obvious example in psychology. When actions that used to produce positive consequences suddenly no longer do, there is an initial increase of that same action in frequency and intensity, and then a series of new and highly variable actions of all kinds. This effect is so predictable that practitioners know, for example, to tell parents when they stop reinforcing their child's undesirable actions to expect this "extinction burst" and to see it as a sign of progress. You can see why evolution would establish changes like this. If doing things to get food suddenly no longer works, the animal that survives will likely be the one that quickly finds new ways forward. If needed variation is artificially restricted—if a person becomes psychologically rigid—pathology is likely to follow.

Selection: Selection means the ability for certain variants to be picked out over others. Typically, they are selected based on the apparently helpful consequences they produce (such as outright survival in the case of genetic evolution). Because short-term consequences can conflict with long-term consequences, however, when dealing with psychopathology often the problem is that psychological adjustments can be adopted that lead to short-term gains and long-term pains. In the context of clinical psychology, a focus on selection often means helping the client to notice ways of being and doing that help or hinder their mental health or positive life trajectories, particularly over the long term, and to choose those that help. For example, a practitioner might ask a client with a pattern of avoidance of social anxiety to record their thought, feelings, and overt actions and to notice how accepting or turning down a social invitation plays out over time, such as a "No, I'm too busy" that leads to relief, followed by depressed mood, negative self-concept, and further social withdrawal.

Retention: Retention means that an individual, group, or culture repeats and strengthens selected variants over time such that they become full-grown habits or customs. In genetic evolution, selected variants are retained physically in DNA. Something like that happens in psychology too when action patterns result in changes in gene expression through epigenetics, changes in the brain based on neural connectivity, and the like. Typically in psychology, however, positive changes are retained by practice, by building larger patterns, and by social-psychological or environmental support. There is a "use it or lose it" quality to most new habits. New learning is also more likely to be retained if it is linked to preexisting habits or customs—what is sometimes called a "broaden and build" strategy. Arranging for social or environmental nudges can also help. Examples of retention strategies abound in applied work: homework, public posting of progress in habit change, keeping track of "streaks," programming positive "nudges," forming a social group to change habits together, and so on.

Context: Context refers to the situational and historical circumstances or intervention goals that affect which behaviors an individual or group selects and retains. For example, some new forms of emotional expression may take hold only if an individual deploys this expression in the context of a loving relationship. Concerns over natural contingencies, cultural fit, connection with religious faith commitments, flexible workplaces, a supportive environment, and so on are all typical ways that practitioners speak of context in an evolutionary sense.

Dimension: Dimension refers to which particular strands of events individuals are selecting and retaining. In the psychological domain, these include affect, cognition, attention, self, motivation, and overt behavior, but dimensions exist in other levels as well.

Level: Level means the degree of organization and complexity of the targets of selection processes. Psychological events involve the whole organism acting within a context that is considered both historically and situationally. But at the biophysiological, genetic, and epigenetic level, selection occurs sub-organismically; and at the sociocultural level, it occurs between dyads and increasingly larger groups and their established rules and customs. Physical abilities and disabilities, diet, exercise, sleep, and measures of biological functioning through brain imaging, genetic, and epigenetic factors are examples of the former; the therapeutic relationship, social support, and interactions with couples/family/friends are examples of the latter.

VRSCDL features can be applied in a robust evolutionary account to any or all of Tinbergen's four key evolutionary questions (Tinbergen, 1963): how the *function* of variants alters adaptation; how these variants emerge and are retained over time in their evolutionary *history*; how these variants *develop* within the lifetime of the organism; and how specific external and internal *mechanisms* combine to produce particular phenotypes, physical or behavioral.

APPLYING EVOLUTIONARY CONCEPTS TO A META-MODEL

We can combine these key concepts of evolution into an "Extended Evolutionary Meta-Model." The EEMM allows us to classify therapeutic processes of change and to consider their integration. The term "meta-model" refers to a model that can incorporate a number of specific models—a model of models.

We can classify processes of change in intervention science into six key psychological dimensions (affect, cognition, attention, self, motivation, and overt behavior), nested into two additional levels of selection (biophysiological and sociocultural). And in each of these dimensions and levels, variation, selection, retention, and context are central (or to use terms that are more familiar to practitioners, each of these dimensions and levels involves processes related to change, function, habits or patterns, and fit and support). Finally, these processes can be adaptive or maladaptive, either helping or hindering mental health and prosperity.

The truth is, therapists already talk in terms of variation, selection, retention, and context: They seek changes that work well for the person (variation and selection), which are built into habits that fit their situation (retention and contextual fit). They apply this to specific dimensions of psychological development (affective, cognitive, behavioral, attentional, motivational, and so on), and they focus on different levels of analysis and the interactions of change processes.

By combining all six evolutionary concepts, we have a broad meta-model for the exploration of adaptive and maladaptive change processes. It organizes multidimensional, multilevel change processes and the specific models that organize them into a larger coherent set called the Extended Evolutionary Meta-Model (see figure 3.2).

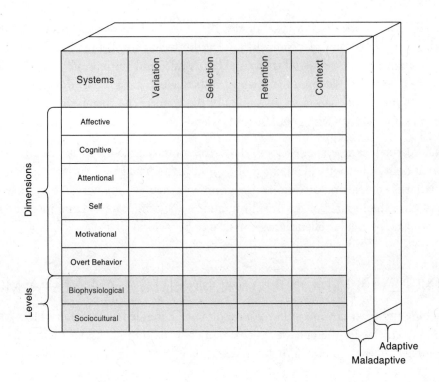

Figure 3.2 The Extended Evolutionary Meta-Model

(copyright Steven C. Hayes and Stefan G. Hofmann)

The top six rows of the EEMM are dimensions of development at the individual level, nested within the two levels in the bottom two rows. Each dimension and level can be examined in terms of variation and selective retention in context. Different "stacks" (labeled "Maladaptive" and "Adaptive") can be created of processes that lead to pathology and those that lead to health. This diagram is a "meta-model" of change processes based on the synthesis that is afforded by modern multidimensional, multilevel evolutionary accounts. Hence, it is called the Extended Evolutionary Meta-Model.

The EEMM is meant not so much as a prescriptive guide but as a common language in which to consider and compare models of change processes. Unlike a formal model, a meta-model can accommodate any specific model that addresses a reasonable range of dimensions, levels, and columns, whether behavioral, cognitive, psychodynamic, humanistic, or other.

This multidimensional and multilevel meta-model approach also suggests whether particular PBT models are sufficiently broad and coherent. If entire rows or columns or stacks are missing in a given model, this suggests that the underlying model is too limited in the identification of change processes in the missing areas. Conversely, if there are several competing models that are reasonably comprehensive, the relative conceptual clarity of the EEMM approach may refine and enhance their empirical comparison.

Action Step 3.1   Explore a Dimension

Let's return to one of the problem areas in your own life. Consider the six dimensions of the EEMM (affect, cognition, attention, self, motivation, and overt behavior), and select one of them that you suspect is relevant to your problem area but that you have not yet exhaustively explored. Select just one dimension—we will get to the others later on in the book.

Now write a few sentences about what seems typical for you in this dimension in your problem area. Are there actions, reactions, or patterns that tend to repeat? Are there any that seem old, familiar, or unhelpful? Find the most common pattern and write about it.

Next, see if you can remember times when you dealt with the dimension you picked inside your problem area in a more effective way than is typical for you. Describe one or two examples of more effective ways of responding.

By way of explanation, the two questions above are about exploring inflexibility and occasions of healthy variation inside the dimension you have chosen. Problem areas tend to have dominant patterns that are not working well but nevertheless tend to repeat. That is what is meant by "inflexibility." If you know about times when you do a better job, then you are seeing indications of "healthy variation." We will use that concept throughout the book.

Example

Dimension: Self

Pattern Inside This Dimension: I feel like a complete loser. Like my achievements are not great enough, and who I am as a person is not good enough. When I get rejected by other people, it is confirmation that I'm not good enough. When I notice I do my best to entertain others, it is again confirmation that I'm not good enough (or else I would not have to try so hard). And when I retreat and go home, yet again, I decide for myself that I'm not good enough.

Example of Responding More Effectively: I was playing volleyball with a friend and his acquaintances. They were all very attractive, and I noticed nervousness and insecurity coming up. But instead of giving in to my fear and labeling myself a loser, I stopped and asked myself what is important right now. The answer was clear: spending quality time with my friend and enjoying myself. As a result, my whole focus shifted, and I could better let go of this idea that I'm not good enough.

How Healthy Variation Applies: My rigid pattern is resorting to self-blame and either trying to prove my self-worth or escaping the uncomfortable situation entirely. One positive variant is refocusing on what truly matters, allowing me to stay in contact with others, without resorting to proving myself.

REVISITING MEDIATION

As you will see, even though the EEMM yields cells, it is a mistake to think of processes of change as inhabiting only specific cells, or even entire rows. Take a process like "attachment." It is a process that occurs between people, so it resides at a sociocultural level to a degree, but it has a psychological impact (such as the affective impact of, say, a relationship that fosters "secure attachment"). That affective impact might in turn select other processes of change (e.g., being less judgmental of others might foster secure attachments and their positive emotional impact). Some processes at the psychological level involve all six psychological dimensions at once. An example is the psychological flexibility model that underlies acceptance and commitment therapy (ACT), which contains six subprocesses, one for each of the six psychological dimensions.

The EEMM looks like a categorical model—for example, there is an "adaptive stack" and a "maladaptive stack"—but in reality, adaptation is probabilistic and dimensional. The field of mental health has divided the world into "psychopathology" and everything else, but life as it is lived is hardly that categorical. Thus, while this more categorical view of the EEMM can be useful, it is important not to think of the EEMM as a kind of "periodic table" designed to sort processes of change into a multidimensional grid. Rather, it shows key functions that clinicians need to think about as they view the individual through the lens of a multidimensional and multilevel evolutionary account.

Waddington's (1953a, 1953b) famous epigenetic landscape can be modified to express the more dynamic and interactive nature of what we are actually arguing. Figure 3.3 shows four "bundles" of biophysiological, psychological, and sociocultural processes and their contextual determinants. All of these processes and contextual features are elastic and interrelated, altering the course of human functioning in an interactive and probabilistic fashion across the life span. That is shown in this visual metaphor by the way that changes in the top surface area modify the probabilities of a particular route followed by the rolling ball, as a metaphor for variation and selective retention modifying the "route" of a human life.

As this physical metaphor emphasizes, no single dimension or level of organization can be said to be the "real cause" of human action and development. That does not mean that some dimensions are not more important than others in particular ways or particular situations. For example, attentional flexibility may be key to maintaining the contextual sensitivity of particular psychological processes; clear motivation may be key for selection of other such processes; overt behavioral habits for retention; and so on. Thus, in the EEMM, the functions noted by the columns in any given row (i.e., in any evolving dimension or level) may be satisfied by processes in another row. For example, greater emotional openness may be selected and retained because it affords greater social intimacy and alliance, cognitive flexibility may be selected and retained because it empowers effective work behaviors, and so on.

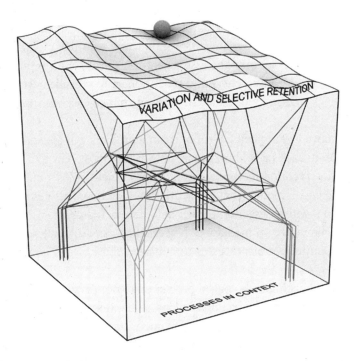

Figure 3.3 A model of how context and processes of change alter the conditions of variation and selective retention that impact human development. The four "bundles" of processes of change represent contextual, psychological, biophysiological, and sociocultural features.

Copyright by Steven C. Hayes and Stefan G. Hofmann. Drawn by Esther M. Hayes. Used by permission.

Thus, from the very beginning it is best to think of the EEMM as a system that helps practitioners and researchers think through how processes of change work and interact with other change processes, more so than a kind of sorting scheme, as if processes of change are pieces of mail to be placed in EEMM mailboxes.

Because our approach to the construction of a process-based alternative to the DSM or ICD has been largely empirical, we can only broadly characterize where this approach is taking us. Consider the following six mediators, each of which we identified in the first dozen studies of that large meta-analysis of therapy mediators we referred to earlier and that we will review in chapter 8: change in obsessive beliefs, cognitive defusion, mindful awareness, change in intrusive thoughts, anxiety sensitivity, and frequency of mindfulness practice. These six concepts apply easily to cognitive, attentional, and affective dimensions. With the exception of the last concept, each is focused on fostering healthy variation. Mindful awareness and anxiety sensitivity carry with them issues of positive and negative contextual sensitivity; frequency of mindfulness practice addresses a retention process in the form of habit formation. It is not hard to place virtually all known mediators in the EEMM.

As we use the EEMM with identified mediators, we see that most of the rows contain several processes to consider. *Moderators,* and dynamical or interactive features, modify how change processes link dimensions, levels, or columns. The assessment tools used for each process will provide a preliminary form of assessment for researchers and practitioners to consider. At that point, we can consider the degree to which existing models of therapeutic change can bear upon a coherent summary of these processes.

Single processes are moved by a specific form of treatment. This will also produce a list of interventions to move processes in each cell. Thus, we are able to link most cells to a variety of measures, processes of change, and intervention methods or treatment kernels, at least broadly.

All other things being equal, models that efficiently cover more of this matrix will be more useful; those that cover less of it will be less useful. Even before we can present a fully organized empirical account of the world's literature on mediation, however, we can still explore what such a system might yield. Even with a limited set of processes to consider, the EEMM approach suggests a way forward.

In this process-based approach, psychological problems are not person-invariant expressions of a latent disease. Instead, we understand psychopathology as context-specific problems in variation, selection, and retention that can occur in a variety of dimensions and levels. This is the core idea of the Extended Evolutionary Meta-Model, which we base on evolutionary science, adapted to psychopathology and psychotherapy.

Because we need to link processes of change to the individual level, a good place to begin in process-based diagnosis is to link identified problems by using a complex network approach to foster a functional analysis of an individual's presenting problems. We can then apply the EEMM framework while considering all relevant past and present contributing factors, such as early life history, attachment styles, traumas, medical issues, beliefs, habits, and so on. We think of treatment as a dynamic change of the complex network from maladaptation to adaptation.

THE TEN STEPS OF PROCESS-BASED FUNCTIONAL ANALYSIS AS A NEW FORM OF DIAGNOSIS

The EEMM combined with network analysis provides a structure for a treatment-relevant approach to process-based diagnosis. We can use these tools to organize a new form of *process-based functional analysis,* which will guide an approach to diagnosis with treatment utility based on known processes of change. It has the following ten steps:

1. Select a theory or model within which to conduct treatment-relevant process-based diagnosis, focusing on models that are reasonably comprehensive as considered within the EEMM and that best fit your setting, population, and background.

2. Relying primarily on the client's report of the central problems or unmet aspirations, identify potentially relevant characteristics of the individual client, their behavior and subjective

experiences, and the context in which they occur via broad assessment organized by the EEMM and informed by the specific model chosen. Make sure this preliminary case description touches on both relevant strengths and weakness in the client's repertoire.

3. Considering the client's goals, organize the network of features of the case description into known change processes and moderators of these processes, expressed both in terms of origin and especially in terms of maintaining conditions. Focus in particular on self-amplifying relations and subnetworks within the network and rely, wherever possible, on empirically established relationships at the individual client level.

4. Add measures of process and outcomes as needed. Gather additional information that will inform the preliminary functional analysis, adding repeated measurement data on the hypothesized primary processes of change if at all possible.

5. Based on that data, reconsider the network, including modifications that emerge in light of nomothetic prototypes drawn from previous idiographic functional analytic work. Organize the network into an integrative, process-based account of the development and maintenance of the maladaptive network. This account is the functional analysis of the case. It is the process-based diagnosis.

6. Consider how to perturbate the dominant features of the network expressed in process-based terms, either directly or indirectly, but make particular consideration of changes that are available, known to respond to intervention, likely to be retained, likely to alter the idiographic functional relations within the maladaptive parts of the client network, and likely to enter idiographically, self-amplifying features of a new adaptive network.

7. Considering the therapeutic context and relationship, select a series of intervention kernels or methods that are most likely to perturbate the network in that fashion.

8. Intervene while continuing to repeatedly measure key change processes, the therapeutic context and relationship, and progress toward the client's goals. Assess the perturbation of the network and the degree of process-level change.

9. If there is no change or inadequate change at the process level, recycle to earlier steps. Normally go back to step 2 or 3, but in some cases, reconsider the EEMM-based model selected in step 1. If there is adequate change at the process level, continue to intervene and assess subsequent outcome movement based on expected links between process and outcome and on the client's goal that is being pursued.

10. If outcomes change sufficiently, attempt to nest idiographic analyses of processes, treatment, and outcomes into nomothetic prototypes as cases gather. If outcomes do not change sufficiently, recycle to earlier steps. Normally this would again be step 2 or 3, but in some cases, reconsider the EEMM-based model selected in step 1.

As knowledge of processes of change increases and measures become more sophisticated, many of these steps can become more automated and empirical for practitioners. For example, as automated measures of outcomes or settings (or repeated measures of processes of change) advance, step 2 may become more routine, and steps 3 through 8 may be more driven by big data. In the interim, we have found it useful in process-based training to teach idiographic conceptual network analysis and to then link process-based functional analysis to the EEMM and repeated assessments. In the following chapters, we demonstrate the utility of the EEMM by applying it to individual clinical cases in a step-by-step fashion, focusing initially on only a few rows or columns so that when the entire system is brought together and used, you will feel confident in its application.

CHAPTER 4

The Cognitive, Affective, and Attentional Dimensions

Now that you have an understanding of the Extended Evolutionary Meta-Model (EEMM), over the next few chapters we are going to explore in more detail manageable subsets of the various dimensions and levels of the EEMM as they apply to particular clients. In this chapter, we will meet a client named Maya, who has chronic pain. Chronic pain is unusual because, unlike with many other ailments, most people with chronic pain are likely to experience pain for the rest of their lives. As a result, they often struggle with their condition and find it hard to accept that their pain may never fully go away.

We are going to use Maya's case to walk through the different dimensions of the Extended Evolutionary Meta-Model (EEMM) and show how each dimension is represented within this client. In Maya's case, the dimensions of cognition, affect, and attention stand central, which is why we put the focus in this chapter on these particular dimensions. We will discuss the remaining dimensions of self, motivation, and behavior in the next chapter.

We start with a clinical intake conversation, where the therapist gathers basic information about Maya's situation and the processes at play. Note that the intake conversation is not specifically "process-based," but instead follows the generic structure of a clinical intake conversation. Afterward, we organize the gathered information into a network model and discuss how Maya's case fits into the dimensions of cognition, affect, and attention. We conclude the chapter by organizing all the gathered elements into a functional analysis. In this manner, you will gain a deeper understanding of how the dimensions of cognition, affect, and attention can be represented in a clinical case, how these elements can be structured into a network model, and how this model is then used to inform a functional analysis. Let's begin.

MAYA'S STRUGGLE

Therapist: What brings you here today?

Maya: Well, I was told by a friend from work that you might be able to help. And at this point I'm really at my end. So here I am. I'll try anything.

Therapist: You'll try anything? And how do you think I could help you?

Maya: Isn't that your job? I mean, I've got this constant pain in my back, and sometimes it hurts so much that I can barely get out of bed, let alone go about my day or go to work or anything. I really don't know what to do anymore. It just makes me so angry, and I'm here to find out how you can help me.

At this point we are barely into the conversation, and already we have learned a few important things about Maya. We have learned that Maya is struggling with chronic back pain and that it makes her restrict her activity and avoid going to work. Additionally, we have learned that this situation is a big source of anger for her. If we put what we have just learned into a network model, it would look similar to what we can see in figure 4.1.

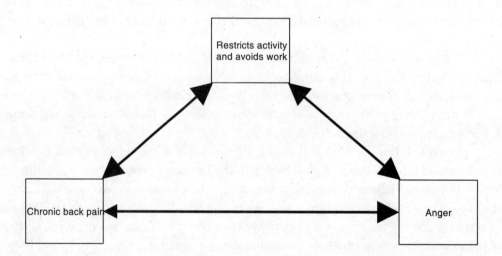

Figure 4.1 Maya's initial network model

Naturally, the factors in Maya's network relate to one another. Maya mentioned that her chronic back pain makes her restrict her activity, but the reverse is likely also true: when she restricts her activity and stays in bed, she is likely to contribute to her back pain (hence the relationship is depicted as a two-way arrow). The same seems true for her level of experienced anger: anger makes Maya restrict herself, and restricting herself feeds into Maya's anger. Lastly, chronic pain feeds into Maya's anger as well. And while the reverse is also true (anger adds to her chronic pain), the influence is weaker from anger toward chronic pain (hence the relationship is depicted as a small arrow). Note that all nodes and their underlying relations might change as we continue to explore Maya's situation.

Therapist: Tell me more about this back pain. How and when did that start?

Maya: About six months ago, I had this injury at work. I'm a nurse and I work in the intensive care unit. And I often have to get supplies for the patients from the storeroom. And so about six months ago, I went to get supplies as usual, and I slipped and fell on my back. And ever since then, I have this excruciating pain that just won't go away.

Therapist: I'm sorry that this has happened to you. How do you normally deal with the pain?

Maya: It's just awful. It hurts so much, and it makes everything so much harder. I mean, I barely go to work anymore. The pain is just always there, and it makes me worry so much, like *What if it stays like this? What if it will never go away?* and so on…

Therapist: So you spend a lot of time thinking about whether the pain will stay.

Maya: Yes. Exactly.

Therapist: And if I would watch you from the outside when you are in the middle of worrying, what would I see you do?

Maya: Not much, I can tell you. I just sit there. Caught up in my own head. And I don't do anything else really.

Therapist: And is this helping you, or is this part of the problem?

Maya: It's definitely part of the problem. When I stay home and do nothing, I just have more time to worry and ruminate. And it just makes me so angry about everything.

We are now deeper into the conversation, and we have learned more about Maya to further inform our network model. For instance, we have learned that Maya sustained her chronic back pain during an injury at work, where she slipped and fell in the storeroom. Furthermore, we have learned that Maya tends to worry a lot about her pain, and that "it might never go away." We have added these new factors as nodes to Maya's network model (see figure 4.2).

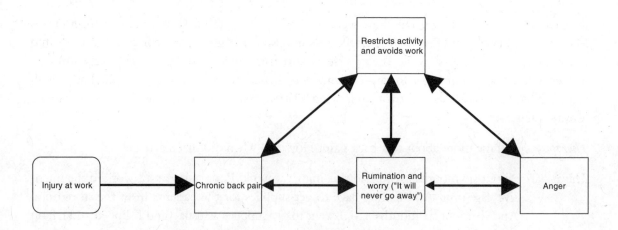

Figure 4.2 Maya's expanded network model

Notice that the new nodes relate to other previously established nodes. For instance, Maya's injury at work has led to her chronic back pain (hence it is depicted as a simple one-way relation). The node "Injury at work" is shaped with round edges because it acts as a moderator (a contextual factor that will not change but modifies how change processes link dimensions, levels, or columns), thus taking on a special role within the network. Furthermore, Maya's rumination and worry about her condition stands central and is connected to several other nodes. Her chronic back pain directly leads her to ruminate and worry, which in turn makes her feel angry. Hence the node "Rumination and worry" stands in between the node "Chronic back pain" and the node "Anger." Notice that anger adds to Maya's tendency to worry, albeit we assume in a smaller way (hence the relation is depicted as a small arrow). Additionally, Maya restricts her activity when she is worrying, which in turn makes her worry even more (hence the relation is depicted as a two-way arrow).

Therapist: And how has your condition affected your work?

Maya: Well, I don't work as much as I used to, because I just cannot. I literally cannot. But it really serves them right.

Therapist: How do you mean?

Maya: I mean, I told my supervisors about this cluttered storeroom again and again. And they just brushed me off, said they are going to do something, and nothing ever happened. The room was a safety hazard, and it was only a matter of time until something happened.

Therapist: So you think the accident was a result of the negligence of your supervisors, and in a way "it shouldn't even have happened."

Maya: Yes. It definitely happened because of my bosses. I mean, it makes me angry just thinking about how unfair it is.

Therapist: And when this sense of unfairness comes up, does it make things easier, or do things become harder?

Maya: I know it doesn't really help. I definitely feel worse then. But I mean, it's true though. It really was their fault, because they didn't take me seriously. I mean, I warned them at least on three occasions!

Bit by bit, we get a better picture of Maya's situation, and we have just learned that Maya blames her bosses for the accident. She had warned them earlier about the cluttered storeroom, and now she feels a sense of unfairness and thinks, *It shouldn't have happened.* This further explains her anger. If we add these new elements to the network model of Maya, it might look similar to figure 4.3.

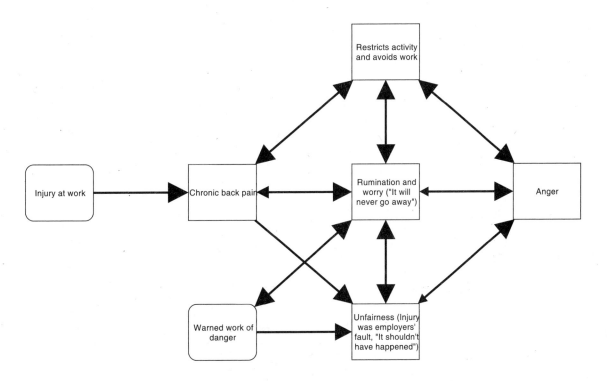

Figure 4.3 Maya's further expanded network model

As usual, these new nodes do not stand alone but are part of a network. Maya had warned her supervisors of the safety hazard, but to no avail, which is why she now feels a sense of unfairness (hence the relation is depicted as another simple one-way arrow). The sense of unfairness, however, is related to several other nodes, where it stands in a self-amplifying loop to Maya's tendency to ruminate and worry, as well as to her anger (although, based on our clinical interview, it appears her sense of unfairness feeds into her anger more than her anger feeds her sense of unfairness—hence the latter relation is depicted with a smaller arrowhead).

As you can see, there are many different factors and processes at play that constitute Maya's situation and that produce, maintain, and facilitate Maya's struggle with chronic pain. We will now begin to sort Maya's experience into the different dimensions of the EEMM, beginning with the dimension of cognition. As we move along with Maya's case, we further explore Maya's situation and uncover additional processes.

THE COGNITIVE DIMENSION

The way clients think about and give meaning to the events in their lives fundamentally shapes their life situation and ability to cope with challenges and difficulties. And Maya is no exception to this truth. Although Maya's chronic pain was not originally a product of her thinking, it is maintained and facilitated by it. That is what makes it especially worthwhile to investigate Maya's cognitions—her thoughts and how she relates to them can give leverage over her struggle with chronic pain. When we take another look at the network model of Maya, we can identify two nodes (highlighted in gray) that fall primarily into the cognitive dimension (see figure 4.4).

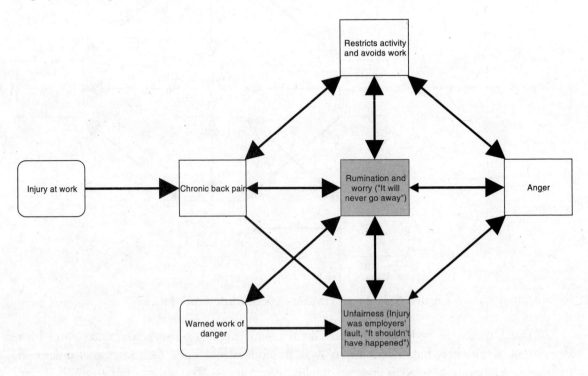

Figure 4.4 The cognitive dimension

In particular, Maya spends a lot of time ruminating and worrying about her life. She ruminates about whether the pain will stay or that it might never go away. Additionally, she seems to have gotten stuck on a sense of unfairness, because she had warned her bosses about the hazard that eventually led to her injury. She blames her bosses for their negligence and says that "it shouldn't have happened."

All of these cognitions eventually add to Maya's anger and reinforce her tendency of activity self-restriction. Naturally, there is more to Maya's story. First of all, several factors are at play in Maya's network that we have not yet uncovered. And we will do so in later parts of the chapter, when we cover the dimensions of affect and attention. Second, although Maya's cognitions exacerbate her struggle in the long term, in the short term they may serve a useful purpose.

Worrying and ruminating might give her a false sense of control, and thus they are psychologically comforting. By engaging her pain in that manner, she might just be able to find an unexpected solution (at least this might be her reasoning, and data suggest that it is a common feature of rumination). Furthermore, entertaining the thought that the injury was "unfair" and that "her bosses are at fault" might be psychologically comforting as well. After all, when the blame is elsewhere, she doesn't have to take responsibility for her own actions or the hard steps she might now need to take to move forward.

In other words, cognitions serve various seemingly useful functions. And while maladaptive thinking patterns might increase long-term suffering, they can be comforting in the short term. Note that all this reasoning is merely speculative and needs to be analyzed more properly with the client in a functional analysis (which we will begin to do later). At this point, it's important to note that cognitive factors that increase long-term suffering often produce seemingly positive or at least helpful short-term results. In fact, this seems to be true of all maladaptive cognitive styles.

The client's need for psychological coherence (in the sense of "this is what is true") can become so dominant that it fosters entanglement with false narratives or unhelpful thinking patterns. Apparent coherence can become the grease on the wheels of thinking in rigid ways that don't fit current needs or provide truly helpful ways forward. Cognitively it is easy for clients dealing with mental health struggles to value form over function, meaning they orient themselves more toward what is "true" rather than what is helpful and adaptive.

Consider the following examples of maladaptive thinking.

Cognitive fusion: Cognitive fusion refers to a thinking style whereby a person identifies with a particular thought (i.e., "fuses" with a thought). From this place, the thought begins to dominate a person's behavior, seeming like an absolute truth or an inevitable command that a person has to obey.

Rumination: Rumination comes in many shapes and forms. A person can ruminate about an event in the past, in search of meaningful lessons, so that this event might not repeat itself. Alternatively, a person can ruminate about the future, in an attempt to avoid a future event, again looking for meaningful answers. In both cases, the person is likely convinced they are doing something productive, while they lose touch with the present moment and exacerbate their pain.

Dysfunctional thinking: Dysfunctional thinking involves expressing negative perceptions of oneself, others, and the world in general. It can undermine a person's sense of self-worth or ability to function effectively. Unfortunately, this type of thinking often becomes automatic, leading to unquestioned interpretations of events, which is why it's often hard to catch such thinking as it happens.

Naturally, there are many more examples of maladaptive cognitive styles, and covering them all would defeat the purpose of this book. What they all have in common is that they tend to be self-amplifying and provide short-term gain at the expense of long-term pain. They are often soothing, providing a false sense of "safety," but with a cost. They restrict thinking and limit the type of thoughts a client is "allowed" to have or entertain. In other words, they limit variation and selection. This often happens automatically, filtering out information that doesn't fit the narrative. Bottom line: It is not irrational for the client to select their maladaptive cognitive style, because it serves a function. It is just not working in their favor.

Unfortunately, it does not help to just point out a client's maladaptive cognitions. Instead, you need to uncover the function of a specific thinking style and offer viable alternative cognitive strategies that allow broader, more flexible thinking, and thus greater variation, selection, and retention. The ways to do so are as plenty as there are different schools of psychotherapy. So instead of covering them all, let's take a look at some examples of adaptive cognitive styles.

Defusion: Defusion is a concept from acceptance and commitment therapy. It describes the process of creating distance between oneself and one's thoughts, where it's possible to have unpleasant and unhelpful thoughts without letting them dominate one's actions.

Cognitive flexibility: Cognitive flexibility refers to the ability to shift one's thinking and attention in response to changing situational demands. A person can thus hold thoughts flexibly and lightly, and can even change previous beliefs or deep-held convictions when they prove to be harmful to the person's goals and well-being.

Reappraisal: Reappraisal refers to the ability to reframe situations and experiences in a way that empowers a person. It is often used to help people who struggle with difficult experiences and help them give new meaning to their anger and pain. Reappraisal is often used in the context of cognitive therapy.

As with the examples of maladaptive cognitive styles, there are many more examples of adaptive cognitive styles. At this point in therapy, it is important to (a) identify the client's cognitive components, and (b) uncover how these components fit into the client's overall pattern. You might find the following guiding questions helpful in sessions with your own clients when you explore problems in variation, selection, and retention in the dimension of cognition. (Note: we will provide guiding questions such as these in several chapters; these can be downloaded from the website for this book, http://www.newharbinger.com/47551.)

Guiding Questions – Cognition

Explore problems in variation—What are the thoughts (and strategies for dealing with thoughts) that show up for the client when they are in their struggle? Which ones have become dominant? Is there any sense of rigidity present in particular cognitions (e.g., dominant "schemas" or repetitive negative thinking) or forms of adjustment to them (e.g., treating them as all literally true)?

Explore problems in selection—Which functions do these thought patterns or forms of adjustment to thoughts serve? Begin with dominant, repetitive, and maladaptive ones, but then move on to more adaptive thoughts or forms of adjustment, however infrequently they make occur.

Explore problems in retention—How do these dominant thought patterns and forms of adjustment maintain and facilitate the client's problems in the network model? In the case of thoughts and adjustment patterns that are adaptive, why are they not retained when they occur? What other features of the network are interfering with retention of gains that may occasionally occur?

Action Step 4.1   Cognition

Let's return to a problem area you identified in your own life in previous chapters. In the "guiding questions," we are asking directly about variation, selection, and retention issues in the area of cognition. See if you can apply the three sets of guiding questions above to the domain of cognition in your own problem area. Write a paragraph about each.

Example

Problems in variation: Thoughts that show up in the middle of my struggle are *I'm embarrassing myself, They won't like me, I just don't have it in me, What am I even doing?* Even though there is a small part of me that knows that this is all just my inner dictator, in the moment it feels like the inevitable truth.

Problems in selection: These thoughts might prevent me from being rejected by others—by rejecting myself first. The alternative, more adaptive thoughts serve to prevent me from rejecting myself and help me stay in touch with what matters to me, namely being present in social situations, potentially building important relationships.

Problems in retention: When I reject myself first, I cannot experience getting accepted as I am—either by myself or by others. The thought *Others will not like me* remains unchallenged, because I do not show my real self to others in the first place. Alternative, adaptive thoughts are available but hard to reach because fear diminishes their believability.

THE AFFECTIVE DIMENSION

The way clients feel about their situation, as well as how they deal with their emotions in general, fundamentally shapes their condition and ability to cope with their problems. Maya's central emotional reaction is her anger, which is influenced by a whole array of other factors.

For instance, we have uncovered that Maya often worries about whether her back pain will ever go away, that she often gets stuck on a sense of unfairness over the workplace accident, and that she tends to restrict her activity and avoids going to work—all of which adds to her anger. However, as we will see, there is more to it. In the subsequent conversation segment, the therapist uncovers an additional factor that belongs in the dimension of affect.

Therapist: You mentioned you often restrict yourself when your pain and anger become too much. And you just said that it's not really helping, and yet you continue doing it, right? So what would you say is good about staying home? If you had to find a reason, what would you say?

Maya: Well, at least I don't get into any more accidents. I'm actually scared of reinjuring myself. I'm afraid of what it might do to my body. And next time, I might end up needing a wheelchair, or even worse.

Therapist: And so your mind says, *It's better to stay home. Just to be safe.*

Maya: Yes, exactly.

Therapist: And are there situations when this fear of reinjuring yourself gets worse? When do you feel it the most?

Maya: Well, it comes up almost anywhere. I used to be especially scared when I thought about returning to work, but now this fear shows up when I get into the supermarket, or even when I get out of the shower or out of bed. I feel my back pain, and I'm immediately scared.

We have just learned a crucial new element that we can add to Maya's network model. We have learned that Maya is scared of reinjuring herself and—as a result—limits her own activities. This fear seems to not be bound to a specific environment but comes up whenever Maya gets in contact with her chronic back pain. If we add this new element to Maya's network model (and highlight the nodes that belong in the dimension of affect), it might look similar to what we can see in figure 4.5.

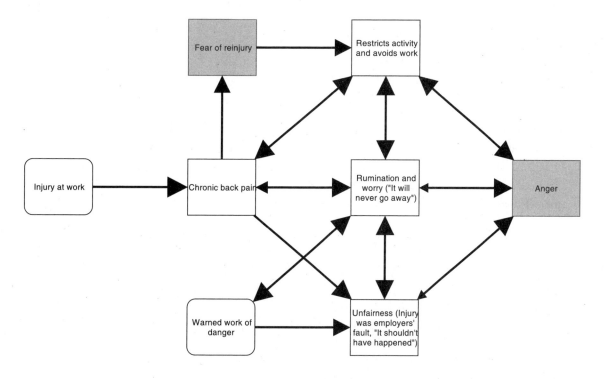

Figure 4.5 The affective dimension

As you can see, the two factors that belong in the dimension of affect are "Fear of reinjury" and "Anger." Neither are yet "processes of change"—they are merely affective events. But these events sustain relationships with other events, and these relationships, or "functions," are processes. Both of these affective factors goad Maya to take ineffective action (i.e., "Restricts activity and avoids work"). This ineffective action of avoiding her fear in turn reinforces her emotional response, thus creating a self-reinforcing cycle, and this entire cycle might be described as a process of change (we will address what to call it later). When Maya restricts her activity, she worsens her chronic pain, which in turn makes her more scared of reinjuring herself. Likewise, when Maya restricts her activity, she may feel more anger because noticing she is not doing things that matter to her will remind her of the cost of the injury.

Maladaptive affective styles show up in all shapes and forms. It's important to note that they may refer to negative emotions (e.g., fear, sadness, boredom, jealousy) but are more specifically about the way a person *relates* to their emotions, "positive" or "negative," and the roles that they have. In other words, the position an emotion takes within the network—the functional role it has—is much more telling than the emotion itself. For instance, there is nothing inherently wrong with being scared of something, unless this fear begins to dominate a person's life and lead to actions that are not adaptive. In Maya's case, her fear of reinjury makes her restrict her activity to the point that it limits her life options and paradoxically worsens her chronic pain—and it is this unwanted self-amplifying process of change that characterizes her fear, and her way of dealing with it, as maladaptive. The goal then is not necessarily to eliminate the negative emotion (e.g., fear, sadness, boredom, jealousy), but to shift its function. In other words, network thinking encourages a focus on how a person is dealing with their negative emotions within the network of their life.

Consider the following examples of maladaptive affective processes.

Experiential avoidance: Experiential avoidance refers to an affective regulation style whereby a person attempts to avoid affective and other internal experiences, even though doing so creates harm in the long term. Experiential avoidance is often motivated by offering short-term relief from discomfort, thereby maintaining the behavior as well as exacerbating the struggle with the object of avoidance.

Shame: Shame is an uncomfortable, self-conscious emotion whereby a person evaluates their own self in a negative way. It often leads the person to withdraw from the situation that has caused or triggered feelings of shame or to believe that they are incapable of being trusted. Shame often comes with feelings of anger, mistrust, fear, powerlessness, vulnerability, and worthlessness. Considered just as an emotion, shame may have a time and place, but because it includes a hidden sense of "I'm bad," it tends to lead to rigidity and cognitive distortion.

Loneliness: Loneliness is an uncomfortable emotional response to perceived social isolation. Purely as an emotion it is not necessarily toxic, but it can self-amplify if it connects to a sense of unworthiness, being unlovable, or other habitual behavioral, cognitive, or self-perception patterns that lead to social isolation or chronic feelings of loneliness even in the presence of caring people.

As with maladaptive thinking styles, there are many more examples of maladaptive affective styles, and it is beyond the scope of this book to cover them. Their common feature is that they tend to be a reaction to a client's circumstances, and they goad the client toward ineffective action patterns in various dimensions. These patterns often have a self-soothing aspect, removing discomfort in the short-term while maintaining pain in the long-term, thus creating a context-insensitive and self-amplifying maladaptive affective style.

As with cognition, it does not suffice to merely point out maladaptive affective processes. Instead, you need to uncover the function of a specific affective process and offer viable alternative strategies that allow broader, more flexible feeling, and thus greater variation. Let's take a look at some examples of more adaptive affective styles.

Acceptance: Acceptance describes the process of allowing unwanted private experiences (e.g., thoughts, feelings, physical sensations, and other internal experiences) to come and go without any unnecessary attempts to change their form or frequency, rather just to learn from their occurrence. Acceptance is not an end in itself but rather a means toward learning from emotional experience and channeling that into more effective action.

Self-compassion: Self-compassion is the ability to extend compassion toward one's self in instances of perceived inadequacy, failure, or general suffering. Self-compassion entails being warm toward oneself when encountering pain, recognizing that suffering is part of the shared human experience, and being aware and accepting of one's own emotions.

Hopefulness: A posture of "hopefulness" is more than a narrowly focused emotion—though it has a strong affective component that reflects an optimistic state of mind, based on an expectation of positive outcomes in one's life or the world at large. Hope can be a reaction to crisis, opening a person up to new creative possibilities.

As with the examples of maladaptive affective styles, there are many more examples of adaptive affective styles. We will list some of the most common ones in chapter 8, based on a vast review of the literature we are conducting. At this point in therapy, it is important to (a) identify the client's relevant affective factors, and (b) uncover how these factors fit into the client's overall pattern. You might find the following guiding questions helpful with your own clients when you explore problems in variation, selection, and retention in the dimension of affect.

Guiding Questions – Affect

Explore problems in variation—What are the emotions and strategies for adjusting to them that show up for the client when they are in their struggle? Which ones have become dominant? Is there any sense of rigidity present in particular emotional patterns and/or forms of adjustment to them (e.g., a restricted range of affect, dominant emotion regulation strategies)?

Explore problems in selection—Which functions do these emotions and patterns of responding to emotions serve? Begin with dominant, repetitive, and maladaptive ones, but then move on to adaptive forms, however infrequently they may occur.

Explore problems in retention—How do these dominant patterns of emotion and adjustment to emotion facilitate the client's problems in the network model? In the case of emotions and adjustment to emotions that are adaptive, why are they not retained when they occur? What other features of the network are interfering with retention of gains that may occasionally occur?

Action Step 4.2   Affect

We will return to the same problem area you chose in Action Step 4.1, but we'll now address emotions and patterns of responding to emotions.

See if you can apply the three sets of "guiding questions" above to the affective domain in your problem area. Write a short paragraph about each.

Example

Problems in variation: Fear, anxiety, and nervousness always show up when I enter a conversation with others (especially strangers, attractive people, and authorities). These emotions become stronger when I actually talk to them. It always happens the same way.

Problems in selection: The fear signals me that something is dangerous and I might get hurt. By having these fears and removing myself from the situation, I can avoid getting hurt. No matter how irrational this seems, the logic holds true in the moment in my mind.

Problems in retention: When I escape a situation because of fear, I never experience the reality that there is nothing to be scared about. I don't experience the fact that getting rejected doesn't hurt nearly as much as I imagine it will. As a result, the fear persists. And even more, the nervousness may even grow stronger the more consistently I escape. After all, if the situation wasn't truly scary, I wouldn't have to escape in the first place.

THE ATTENTIONAL DIMENSION

The way clients direct and shift their focus on external and internal experiences fundamentally shapes their situation. So far, we have uncovered several factors that capture and direct Maya's attention, ultimately facilitating and maintaining her struggle. For instance, Maya often ruminates and worries about her chronic back pain, and she tends to get stuck on a sense of unfairness over her injury (since she attributes the accident to her bosses). These factors, while belonging to the dimension of cognition, also let us know where Maya directs and focuses her attention. In other words, Maya focuses a lot on her pain, which in turn reinforces other parts of the network.

Therapist: Can I ask you to do a little exercise with me? It only takes ten seconds, but it might be insightful.

Maya: Yes, sure.

Therapist: Great. In a moment, I will set the timer for ten seconds, and during that time, I want you to count everything you can see in this room that is brown. And when I say stop, I want you to close your eyes. Ready?

Maya: Yes, I'm ready.

Therapist: Alright, go! Look for brown, look for brown, look for brown *(waits ten seconds)*. And stop. Now, with your eyes closed, please tell me everything you saw that is red!

Maya: *(chuckles)*

Therapist: You can open your eyes again. It's difficult isn't it?! It's a silly little exercise, but it shows that whatever we focus on will take center stage in our mind, while we miss out on a lot of other things around us.

Maya: I get it, but what does this have to do with me?

Therapist: Well, when you are in the middle of your struggle, what do you focus on?

Maya: Hm, I'm not sure. I would think my back pain. And how hard and unfair this whole mess is, and how angry it makes me.

Therapist: And when you focus on your pain like this, does it get better or worse?

Maya: I can definitely feel it more when I fully focus on it.

Therapist: And how about these thoughts of "this is unfair" and "it shouldn't have happened"? Do these thoughts get bigger, smaller, or stay the same when you focus on them?

Maya: They definitely get bigger. It feels so heavy sometimes.

Therapist: I understand. And what would you say, when are you most likely to focus on your pain?

Maya: I think when it gets really hard for me, and when I get caught up in my own head. You know, it feels like there's nothing else then.

In this last segment, we have learned that Maya focuses a lot on her pain, and that this focus tends to make things even harder for Maya. She then experiences more back pain, ruminates more, and gets even more stuck with her sense of unfairness. Additionally, she adds to her anger. Lastly, Maya mentioned that she focuses more on her pain when she feels the full weight of her anger and when she gets stuck on her sense of unfairness. Thus, there are multiple self-reinforcing loops, giving Maya's attentional style a central role in her network. If we add this new element—"Attention to pain," highlighted in gray—to Maya's network model along with its relations to other factors, it might look similar to what we can see in figure 4.6.

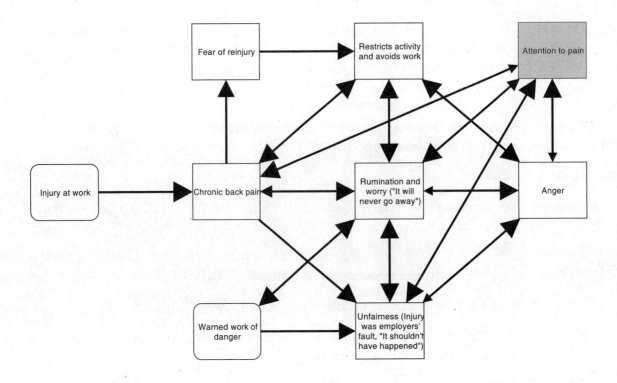

Figure 4.6 The attentional dimension

Maya's focus on her pain facilitates a whole range of other factors and processes that ultimately maintain and exacerbate her ailment. As such, it is central not only to her struggle, but also to her solution. By merely changing Maya's attentional style, she is likely to experience a shift in adjacent factors and processes as well. In subsequent chapters, we will further address what treatment might look like for Maya.

It is not uncommon for clients—especially those dealing with chronic pain—to rigidly focus on their pain. Nonetheless, there are many more variants of maladaptive attentional styles. It's important to note that it's not just the object of the client's attention but the manner and frequency that determines whether an attentional style is maladaptive or not. For instance, a client can focus on their pain from a curious, detached perspective. In this way, the object remains the same (namely pain), but the manner is different (open instead of rigid), thus changing how the attentional style affects other nodes within the network. We consider those attentional styles maladaptive that facilitate processes that work against the client's deeper interests. Consider the following examples of maladaptive attentional styles.

Rigid attention: Rigid attention refers to an attentional style whereby a person gets stuck on a specific thought, emotion, physical sensation, or other internal experience. The object of attention becomes the main focus, and the person experiences difficulty letting go of this focus—even at the cost of not accomplishing other long-term objectives.

Scattered focus: Scattered focus refers to an attentional style whereby a person experiences difficulty maintaining their focus on a particular object (whether external or internal) for a longer period of time. This inability to sustain attention often makes it difficult to attain long-term objectives.

Excessive attending to the past/future: Excessive attention to the past or the future refers to an attentional style whereby a person frequently guides their attention to events outside of the present moment, at the cost of not attaining objectives in the here and now. A person can excessively focus on events in the past, and thereby exacerbate their pain, or they can excessively focus on a possible future, and thereby exacerbate their fear. These can be thought of as the attentional aspect of rumination and worry.

Again, there are many more examples of maladaptive attentional styles, which we won't cover here. They all direct a person's attention in a psychologically comfortable way that interferes with healthy development. The focus can be on sources of psychological pain, thereby keeping the mind engaged. Alternatively, the focus can be deliberately away from sources of pain, like "putting one's head in the sand." In both cases, the attentional style removes immediate discomfort in the short term while maintaining discomfort in the long term, thus reinforcing the maladaptive attentional style and creating a self-reinforcing loop. Again, it is not irrational for the client to engage in a maladaptive attentional style. It is just not workable in the long term.

As with maladaptive cognitions and affect, it does not suffice to merely point out maladaptive attentional styles. Instead, you need to uncover the function of a specific attentional style and to offer viable alternative strategies that allow broader, more flexible feeling, and thus greater variation. There are numerous ways to do so; instead of covering them all, let's take a look at some examples of adaptive attentional styles.

Mindfulness: Mindfulness describes an attentional style whereby a person is engaged and attentive to events unfolding in the present moment. The person observes these events in an intentional (i.e., self-directed) and nonjudgmental way, meaning all experiences that show up in the present moment are valid and are to be observed.

Acting with awareness: Acting with awareness is an attentional style whereby a person is in contact with their experience in the here and now and takes conscious actions that are in alignment with their goals or intentions.

Attentional flexibility: Being able to narrow or broaden one's attention, or to hold or shift attention, in a flexible, fluid, and voluntary way is a meta-cognitive skill that can be trained and learned and that can be useful in dealing with a wide variety of clinical situations.

As with the examples of maladaptive attentional styles, there are many more examples of adaptive attentional styles. At this point in therapy, it is important to (a) identify the client's attentional components, and (b) uncover how these components fit into the client's overall pattern. You might find the following guiding questions helpful in sessions with your own clients when you explore problems in variation, selection, and retention in the dimension of attention.

Guiding Questions – Attention

Explore problems in variation—Where does the client put their attentional focus when they are in their struggle? Is there any sense of rigidity present in their attentional process (e.g., being unable to maintain a focus or to shift focus from a particular area, being drawn into the interpreted past or imagined future while missing the ongoing present, or being excessively broad or narrow in attentional focus)?

Explore problems in selection—Which functions do these attentional patterns serve within the client's network of events? Begin with dominant and problematic attentional patterns, but then move on to more adaptive attentional patterns that are more flexible, fluid, and voluntary.

Explore problems in retention—How do attentional patterns facilitate the chronic occurrence of client's problems in the network model? Why are more adaptive attentional patterns not retained when they occur? What other features of the network are interfering with a healthy retention of gain?

Action Step 4.3   Attention

Consider the same problem area you have been addressing in this chapter, but now focus on attentional patterns. See if you can apply the three sets of guiding questions above to the attention domain in your problem area. Write a paragraph about each.

Example

Problems in variation: When I'm inside my struggle, I always focus on myself. I focus on my thoughts, my nervousness, and the weird feelings inside my body. I lose touch with what is happening around me.

Problems in selection: I believe I do not want to make any mistakes, and therefore I monitor myself much more in social settings than I would normally do. Additionally, I try to solve the problem of my fear and nervousness by thinking my way out of it, hence I focus on myself yet again.

Problems in retention: By excessively focusing on myself, I play it safe. I miss what is out there, and who knows what I might have missed, had I dared to stop monitoring myself?! The attention on myself gives me a false sense of safety that is never challenged—hence it persists. Putting the focus outside, on the other hand, seems risky, because I might say something stupid.

FUNCTIONAL ANALYSIS OF MAYA

When it comes to a process-based functional analysis, we need to start at the end. Functional analysis is relevant to both originating and maintaining conditions (i.e., those contributing to how a problem came to be, and those contributing to sustaining it), but in both cases "function" refers to a target or goal. In Maya's case, the two primary ends that have been uncovered so far are anger and restriction of activity. Of the two, anger appears to be more central to what has caused Maya to seek treatment, although restriction of activity may well be more key to what is maintaining the chronic pain itself. Given Maya's focus, let's begin with anger as a focus and work backward from there, considering processes that may be involved in fostering and maintaining anger.

When looking for processes of importance, we first focus on possible self-amplifying aspects of the network that could be related to the target. Potentially self-amplifying features will be present when there are double-headed arrows ("edges" in network lingo) or subnetworks that enter into closed loops of three or more nodes. If we begin with anger and work backward, we can look across the three dimensions of the EEMM we have been discussing in this chapter and consider especially those nodes, edges, and subnetworks that might self-amplify in the areas of affect, cognition, and attention. In essence, any of these potentially self-amplifying features can operate as selection and retention mechanisms.

In the cognitive domain, Maya's anger is impacted both by rumination and worry and by the belief that this situation is unfair. And because these relationships are bidirectional in both cases, they alone can self-amplify, regardless of the rest of the network. That likelihood is increased further by the two-way relation between entanglement with thoughts about how unfair this is, and rumination and worry. These three nodes (anger, rumination and worry, thoughts of unfairness) then form a possible self-amplifying loop of entanglement with dysfunctional or catastrophic thinking and rumination through their relationship to anger. Because of their potentially self-amplifying properties, these cognitive processes can become more and more likely, narrowing Maya's cognitive repertoire. If you are ruminating or focusing on unfairness, it means you are also *not* thinking more creatively about your situation. Because Maya is visiting this cognitive style regularly, it becomes well practiced, thus more likely to be retained and less sensitive to context.

As is the case for most cognitive processes, what selects them appears to be their explanatory power and the sense of understanding, coherence, and control they provide. These selective benefits foster a kind of interaction between dimensions of the EEMM. Anger makes sense of rumination and unfairness—for example, an angry reaction is evidence of the very unfairness that Maya is focusing on. These relationships are displayed in Table 4.1.

Table 4.1 Maya's EEMM: Cognition and Affect (Anger)

	Variation	Selection
Cognition	Rumination and dysfunctional thoughts of fairness	Making sense of the past; dealing with the future; social support; anger
Affect	Anger	Focus on the past makes sense of anger

When people ruminate or worry, they commonly believe they will be better positioned to deal with present or future challenges. In fact, that is not what occurs, but the sense that it could be so can serve as a self-sustaining consequence.

It is also possible that expressions of unfairness will be widely supported socially, since warnings of workers indeed are often unfairly ignored, as seems to have happened here. Friends and family will likely fail to distinguish between the rational belief that there may be an unfair process of oppression of the powerless involved on the one hand, and the psychological fact that Maya is becoming so entangled with this core belief that she is almost sacrificing her life to prove that point.

A secondary loop is the relationship of these cognitive processes to avoidance behavior and work absence at the top of the network, as we saw in figure 4.6. When entangled in rumination, Maya is more likely to restrict her behaviors and to avoid work. Not only does this cause further anger, but ironically it is a well-established fact that pain avoidance behaviors (e.g., defensive holding, guarded physical postures) tend to exacerbate back pain itself. These more dominant instances of pain in turn feed the process of cognitive narrowing.

Thus, when we look at the set of nodes in this network, with rumination and worry placed at its center, each of the nodes within that part of Maya's psychological network tends to elaborate and sustain the importance and occurrence of the overall network.

At the affective level, Maya's fear of reinjury also further increases the likelihood of activity restriction and work absence through the process of fear avoidance. And as we have just described, this increases pain further, fostering processes of cognitive narrowing. All of that further increases her anger.

What selects this emotional process initially may be actual reduction of fear in the short term, but it is at the cost of an increase in the impact of this fear in the long run. Thus, as with the cognitive processes, this affective process becomes more likely as it is repeated, not just because it is now a habit, but because the contextual cues that establish this fear (i.e., feeling back pain) may be more likely as a result. Table 4.2 depicts these relationships.

Table 4.2   Maya's EEMM: Cognition and Affect (Fear of Pain; Anger)

	Variation	Selection
Cognition	Rumination and dysfunctional thoughts of fairness	Making sense of the past; dealing with the future; social support; anger; avoidance behavior leads to more pain
Affect	Fear of pain; anger	Focus on the past makes sense of anger; avoidance behavior leads to more pain

The final set of processes—those of attention—locks this network together in a way that makes it both very likely to grow and relatively insensitive to contextual features that might lead to new ways of adjusting to pain. When Maya is feeling angry, her attention returns to her back pain and from there to both her fear of reinjury and her entanglement with dysfunctional thinking styles. When she is attending to these features of her life, she is also *not* attending to other, more adaptive ways she may sometimes handle her pain or think more flexibly. Thus, even if there are seeds of healthy growth in her day-to-day functioning, her rigid attentional focus overwhelms any sensitivity to those opportunities to change. This is depicted in Table 4.3.

Table 4.3   Maya's EEMM: Cognition, Affect, and Attention

	Variation	Selection
Cognition	Rumination and dysfunctional thoughts of fairness	Making sense of the past; dealing with the future; social support; anger; avoidance behavior leads to more pain
Affect	Fear of pain; anger	Focus on the past makes sense of anger; avoidance behavior leads to more pain
Attention	Attention to pain	Attention to pain when feeling anger; attention to pain after thoughts of unfairness; felt pain

In summary, Maya's network model shows an interlocking set of cognitive, affective, and attentional processes (along with overt behavior) that are minimizing healthy variation and adaptive context sensitivity, and that are locked together in a self-sustaining network. Maya, in short, is stuck inside her struggle with chronic pain. And the end result is both poorer behavioral functioning and more anger.

In order to take this analysis to another level, it is important to gather additional information that will inform the preliminary process-based functional analysis. There are more dimensions to explore, which we will cover in the next chapter.

Action Step 4.4   Fill in Your EEMM: Cognitive, Affective, and Attentional Dimensions

Let's return to the problem you identified in your own life. Please draw a partial EEMM based on what you have done in Action Steps 4.1 through 4.3. Fill in the relevant dimensions as they relate to your problem, considering both the variability and selection of maladaptive features. Please note that your problem may not be very well represented in all dimensions. We are skipping the columns for retention and context sensitivity because often these involve features of other dimensions, and thus a partial EEMM may not cover what you need.

| | MALADAPTIVE | |
	Variation	Selection
Cognition		
Affect		
Attention		

Example

	MALADAPTIVE	
	Variation	**Selection**
Cognition	I focus on possible failure far more than on how to succeed.	It gives me the sense that I can control possible problems if I am just vigilant enough. However, it also interferes with my ability to listen and be with people.
Affect	I tend to turn down socially challenging situations that might make me anxious.	I immediately feel better but I also soon fear the next situation even more.
Attention	I watch for signs of impending anxiety that might arise.	I feel safer and less vulnerable, but it interferes with my performance, and when I notice that I feel even more anxious. It feels like I'm on a sick merry-go-round.

CHAPTER 5

The Self, Motivational, and Behavioral Dimensions

In the previous chapter, we learned about Maya, a client with chronic pain, to illustrate the dimensions of cognition, affect, and attention and to begin to consider these psychological dimensions within the Extended Evolutionary Meta-Model (EEMM), which organizes process-based therapy (PBT). In this chapter, we will explore the remaining psychological dimensions of self, motivation, and overt behavior. We will do so using the case of Julie, a client who struggles in her close relationships but is coming in for individual therapy.

Relationship difficulties can be hard to address in individual therapy because their dynamics, by definition, involve more than the individual client. It is not uncommon to have to intervene with only one partner, however. Sometimes the psychological focus of the work warrants that approach—other times work needs to be done with an individual even to progress toward a situation in which the couple *per se* can be the issue.

Let's start with a clinical intake conversation, as the therapist gathers basic information about Julie's situation. As in the previous chapter, the conversation follows the structure of a typical clinical intake, but we will mix in sensitivities from a number of different perspectives in an attempt not to be constrained by any particular psychotherapeutic orientation.

It is important to stay as close as possible to Julie's own subjective report—this is the raw material that serves as the basis of PBT. Asking open-ended questions and using reflective listening provides a clinical on-ramp to ensure that the therapist understands the client's inner world. We will then organize the gathered information into a network model, and then discuss how Julie's case fits into the dimensions of self, motivation, and behavior. We will conclude the chapter by organizing all the gathered elements into a functional analysis.

JULIE'S ISSUE

Therapist: What brings you here today?

Julie: I actually have a pressing issue, but I feel like it's a more general pattern as well. So I was hoping we could talk a little bit about it, and maybe find a solution of some sort to help me get better.

Therapist: Why don't you go ahead and tell me more about this pressing issue.

Julie: Yes, so a little bit of a backstory: My husband is a full-time student and he is about to finish his bachelor's degree and go on with his master's. And I'm a dentist with my own private practice. And as part of my ongoing education, I want to attend an important dental conference, which is occurring at the same time as his finals.

Therapist: Okay.

Julie: When I said that I would be going to this conference, he made a comment of "No, you're not." And today is the deadline to register for the conference, and I have been in anguish about having this conversation with him so I can go.

Therapist: So your husband does not support your wish to attend, and you have been avoiding talking to him about it.

Julie: Yes. I haven't really talked to him about it since he made that comment. And I'm committed to going to the conference. I'm going. But I don't really know how to stand up for myself and tell him I'm going. That's why I have been putting it off.

Therapist: You also mentioned that this might be a general pattern. Would it be fair to assume that this is not the first time you have been putting off difficult conversations?

Julie: Yes, that is true. I never know what to say or how to convince him.

The first few minutes of the conversation already reveal a lot about Julie's situation. We have just learned that Julie is struggling to stand up for herself in front of her husband, who does not support her wish to attend a conference. Furthermore, we have learned that this led Julie to avoid having a difficult conversation with her husband. If we put what we have just learned into a network model, it would look similar to what we can see in figure 5.1.

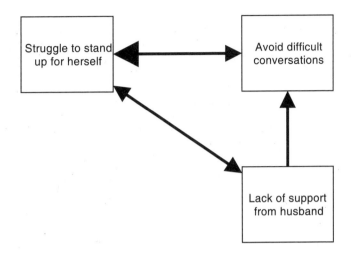

Figure 5.1 Julie's initial network model

Naturally, the factors in Julie's network do not stand in isolation but relate to one another. Julie mentioned that she struggles to stand up for herself, which is why she has been avoiding having a difficult conversation with her husband. However, the reverse is likely also true: because she frequently avoids difficult conversations, she does not get the practice of standing up for herself and thus struggles with it. Chances are that this relation is stronger than the other way around, which is why this relation is depicted as a two-way arrow, with one arrowhead being bigger than the other. Furthermore, she struggles to stand up for herself because she perceives her husband as unsupportive. And here again, the reverse is likely also true: her husband appears to be outright unsupportive, but Julie's history of struggling to stand up for herself makes it easier for him to ignore Julie's wishes, which is why this relation too is depicted as a two-way arrow. Lastly, Julie avoids difficult conversations of all kinds—not just in the service of standing up for herself—and that includes with her husband when he appears unsupportive. We're not sure if that more general pattern of avoiding difficult conversations is inadvertently leading to a lack of support from her husband, so for now we will leave the arrow one headed, but that may well change as we gather more information.

The three factors we have just put into nodes constitute the core of Julie's situation. So far the network consists of only three factors, and yet it is already linked into a positive feedback loop, where the factors relate to each other and exacerbate one another. As we explore the dimensions of self, motivation, and overt behavior, we will continue to explore Julie's case and uncover additional factors and processes that further inform Julie's network model.

THE SELF DIMENSION

The way clients think about themselves and attempt to preserve a certain self-image fundamentally shapes their lives and ability to address problems. This is true for any client, and it is true for Julie. So far into the intake conversation we have uncovered that Julie is struggling to stand up for herself and—as a result—tends to avoid difficult conversations, especially with her husband. We have not yet uncovered originating or maintaining factors behind this pattern. In the subsequent conversation segment, the therapist discovers additional factors in Julie's network model that belong to the dimension of self.

Therapist: You mentioned you struggle to stand up for yourself in difficult conversations with your husband. Do you notice this being a difficulty for you with other people as well?

Julie: I think I have never been really good at it. I often feel shy and timid around others. I definitely notice that I struggle to stand up for myself in general, not just with my husband.

Therapist: When you say that you have "never been really good at it," about how old would you say you were when this first became apparent to you?

Julie: I'm not sure, but pretty young. I don't know, maybe five or six or so?

Therapist: Five or six. That is pretty young. So, you were just a small child.

Julie: Yes.

Therapist: And who would five-year-old Julie need to stand up to?

Julie: I'm not sure...definitely my mother.

Therapist: Your mother?

Julie: Yes. My mother and I often got into each other's faces. She had these ideas of how little girls are supposed to be. I mean, I think we had a good relationship, and we still do. But I wasn't allowed to do much of what I wanted when I was younger, because she had different ideas for me.

Therapist: Can you tell me more about what you mean by "different ideas"?

Julie: Sure. I was always the type of girl to get myself dirty playing outside, and I mostly used to play with boys. And my mom did not really like that. She always told me that "nice girls don't behave like this," and she tried to make me more "girly" in general. This has pretty much continued to this day even. And part of that is I'm supposed to serve others—including her really. What I wanted was not necessarily in the picture.

Therapist: And when you behaved unlike a "nice girl" and acted in your own self-interest, what would your mother say to you?

Julie: Well, she would quickly shut it down. If I didn't do what she wanted, she often told me that I "shouldn't be so selfish."

Therapist: Does that programming still echo into the present in this situation with your husband and thinking about going to the conference? Does "selfish" show up in your mind?

Julie: Yes, I think it does. I really want to go to the conference—I'm going—but once this selfish thought pops up, I get even more nervous about what everybody else will think of me, and it makes me want to retreat into a shell. When it's like this, I easily falter with the tiniest bit of pushback.

Therapist: So when this thought of "I shouldn't be selfish" comes up, along with this feeling of wanting to retreat, you struggle even more to stand up for yourself, and you are even less likely to get into confrontations, did I get that right?

Julie: Yes, pretty much. I just tuck my head in and don't speak up.

We have just learned some crucial new elements that we can add to Julie's network model. We have learned that Julie struggles to stand up not only to her husband, but also to other people. This has been difficult for her ever since she was a young child, when she used to have frequent disputes with her mother about how she should behave. Furthermore, we have learned that her mother tried to mold her into a "nice girl," defining her purpose as one of passive service, while her own needs and preferences were called "selfish." To this day, Julie often feels shy and timid around others—especially when she acts in her own self-interest.

If we add these new elements to Julie's network model (and highlight those nodes that belong in the dimension of self), it might look similar to what we can see in figure 5.2. Note that the node containing Julie's history with her mother has round edges to differentiate it as a contextual factor that will not change but is part of the origin of the issue at hand. As a reminder, in more technical language, these nodes are "moderators."

Julie's history with her mother has fundamentally shaped her current situation and her view of herself. Her mother tried to mold her self-concept in way that has led to struggles to stand up for herself, and led her to feel shy around others (hence both relations are depicted as simple one-way arrows). Furthermore, whenever Julie pushed back or acted in her own self-interest, her mother told her to "not be so selfish." This self-concept had an effect on Julie, so that whenever she intends to act in her own interest, she is quick to think that she is indeed acting "selfishly" and that she should not be doing so (hence the relation is depicted as a one-way arrow). Her intention to not to be "selfish" greatly hinders her ability to stand up for herself and supports her tendency to avoid difficult conversations. Additionally, it fuels her feelings of shyness around others. Not standing up for herself, however, also feeds that self-concept in a notable way, thus the two-headed arrow.

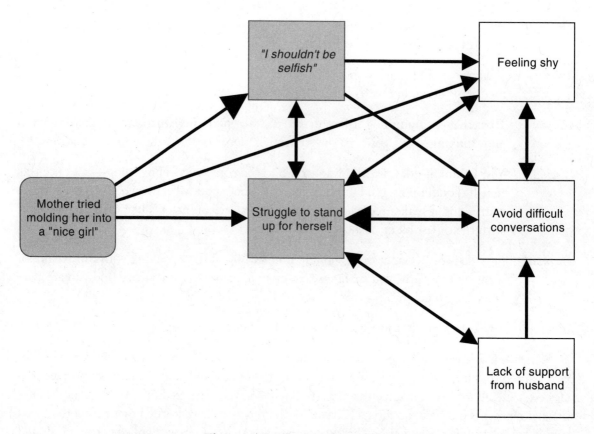

Figure 5.2 The self dimension

It is probably fair to assume that Julie is less likely to enter a confrontation when she is feeling shy, and that her avoidance of difficult conversations in turn further fuels her feelings of nervousness around others (hence this relationship is depicted as a two-way arrow). When she is feeling shy in this way, she struggles even more to stand up for herself, which in turn—yet again—also fuels her feelings of shyness. Although Julie's sense of self and who she is "supposed to be" exacerbates her struggle in the long term, in the short term it serves a purpose. Through her personal history with her mother, Julie might have come to associate acting like a "nice" girl with the feeling of being loved, while associating being more independent with a sense of criticism and possible abandonment. These associations have stuck with Julie to this day, so that she only allows herself to feel loved when she is acting "nice" and denies herself feeling loved whenever she is acting "selfish." Since she was often labeled "selfish" whenever she dared to stand up to her mother, she quickly learned to cave in to other people's demands and wishes and avoid difficult conversations entirely. While Julie's narrative about herself maintains and exacerbates her struggle to stand up for herself, it also creates a psychological safe space where she can feel loved if she behaves "nice."

In other words, again, Julie's narrative about herself and how she is supposed to be serves a useful function. And while it might increase long-term suffering, it may serve to be comforting in the short term.

Note that all this reasoning is merely speculative and needs to be analyzed more properly with the client within the context of a functional analysis (which we will do at the end of this chapter) and empirical evaluations. At this point, it's important to note that all factors that increase long-term suffering often produce short-term results that maintain their role.

Consider the following examples of maladaptive self styles.

Conceptualized self: The conceptualized self is a concept from acceptance and commitment therapy (ACT). It refers to the narrative we create about ourselves—who we are as a person and what we can and cannot do. We use this narrative not only to define ourselves, but also to compare ourselves to others. Unfortunately, as we use this sense of self to evaluate and compare, we tend to allow ourselves to be limited by the content of our narrative.

Event centrality: Event centrality refers to the tendency for traumatic or other specific negative life events to become central in the organization of an individual's identity and narrative life story.

Dissociative identities: Individuals with dissociative identities are unable to integrate life events within a single psychological life course, and instead "split" life into two or more "personalities," each with relatively distinct and disconnected sets of memories, affect, behavior, and thinking style.

These are only some of the many examples of maladaptive self styles. The important point is that all self styles tend to be self-amplifying and provide short-term gain at the expense of long-term pain. They are often soothing, providing a false sense of "safety," but with the cost of capturing a person's sense of self and narrowing it more. They limit the type of thoughts, feelings, and actions a client is "allowed" to have or engage in. In other words, they limit variation and selection. This often happens automatically—information that doesn't fit the narrative gets ignored or is met with a strong inner conflict. The bottom line: It is not irrational for the client to select their maladaptive self style, because it serves a function. It is just not working in their favor.

It does not help to just point out a client's maladaptive sense of self. Instead, you need to uncover the function of a specific narrative and offer viable alternative strategies that allow a broader, more flexible sense of self, and thus greater variation, selection, and retention. Here again, we will take a look at some examples of the numerous ways to do so.

Observing self / Decentering: The self as a point of awareness, or a "decentered" perspective, is part of several clinical approaches. There are many names for this sense of a noticing, witnessing, contextual, decentered, perspective-taking sense of self in which a person experiences themself as an observer, rather than as the content of what is observed. From this point of view, the individual may be able to acknowledge thoughts, feelings, and other internal experiences more freely and flexibly, without attachment to any of them.

Self-worth: Self-worth refers to the inherent worth and value that a person believes they have. This worth is given by nobody but the person themself, although the belief is often influenced by parental upbringing and other environmental factors. A lack of self-worth is often credited as making people behave in self-destructive ways, whereas a high sense of self-worth is assumed to make people act in life-enhancing ways.

Self-efficacy: Self-efficacy refers to the belief people have about their ability to achieve the outcomes they wish to achieve. A high sense of self-efficacy is believed to be underlying high self-esteem, and it is credited as making people act in productive ways. Naturally, a lack of self-efficacy is believed to do the opposite and lead people to behave in unproductive ways.

As with the examples of maladaptive self styles, there are many more examples of adaptive self styles. At this point in therapy, it is important to (a) identify the client's components related to the self, and (b) uncover how these components fit into the client's pattern. You might find the following guiding questions helpful in sessions with your own clients when you explore problems in variation, selection, and retention in the dimension of self.

Guiding Questions – Self

Explore problems in variation—Is there a sense of self, or a self-concept, that shows up for the client when they are in their struggle, or that fails to appear that might be helpful? Is there any sense of rigidity or a lack of healthy variation in the domain of self?

Explore problems in selection—What are the functions of a problematic sense of self? If or when a healthier sense of self or self-concept appears, what functions might it serve?

Explore problems in retention—In the area of self, how do these dominant patterns support, facilitate, or maintain the client's problems in the network model? In the case of a more adaptive sense of self or self-concept, why is it not retained when it occurs? What other features of the network are interfering with retention of gains that may occasionally occur?

Action Step 5.1   Self

See if you can apply the three sets of guiding questions above to the dimension of self in the problem area of yours that you selected to work on. Write a paragraph about each.

Example

Problems in variation: The sense of self that shows up is that *I'm a loser* or *I'm an idiot*, and *I'm not good enough*. These thoughts seem very convincing in the middle of my struggle.

Problems in selection: By denouncing myself first, I protect myself from potential attacks of outsiders. By rejecting myself first, I avoid getting rejected by others.

Problems in retention: My sense of self as a "loser" is never challenged, because I never show up in a way that would allow others to embrace who I am. Instead, this self-perception is reinforced each time I reject myself (i.e., only a loser would think of themself as a loser).

THE MOTIVATIONAL DIMENSION

The client's motivation underlies both their problem development and their possibilities for change. This is true for any client, as it is for Julie. So far into the conversation we have learned what Julie wishes to avoid, namely, getting into confrontation with others and being seen as selfish—either by herself or by others. However, we know little about what actually drives her forward, how she wishes to act, and what she wants to accomplish. In the following conversation segment, the therapist uncovers parts of Julie's underlying motivation.

Therapist: We have talked a bit about what you don't want, that you don't want to be seen as "selfish," and that you wish to avoid difficult conversations. Let's flip this around and look at the other side of things you actually *do* want for yourself.

Julie: Okay, that sounds good to me.

Therapist: You mentioned you are a dentist with your own private practice, right?

Julie: Yes, exactly.

Therapist: Tell me more about your work. How is this going for you?

Julie: Well, it actually is going pretty well. Since my husband doesn't really work yet other than his studies, I'm the sole breadwinner in our relationship. And my practice is doing well, so it's not really a problem. My patients seem to like me, and my schedule is frequently full.

Therapist: Great! So it would be fair to say you have a highly successful career?

Julie: Yes, I think that's fair to say.

Therapist: And what about being a dentist is important for you?

Julie: Well, there's a lot really. I really like my field, and I think I'm pretty good at it too. And I feel like I can help other people, which is very important for me. And I'm being recognized for my work…that's one reason for going to this conference. I mean, some of that programming is probably from my mother to be honest, but I genuinely want to make a positive difference in people's lives.

Therapist: How does your wish to help other people relate to your struggle to stand up for yourself?

Julie: Realistically it helps, but emotionally it's different. When I assert myself, it helps me do what I came to do...but then there is this nagging sense that I'm doing it on the back of other people.

We have just learned new information about Julie, which we can add to her network model. We have learned that Julie is highly successful in her career as a dentist, and as part of her job she values helping other people. She has a genuine motivation of helping others through her work, but because of the overlap with her history in which "helping others" was used to close down her own sense of agency, when she stands up for herself it feels like it's on the "backs of other people" even when it's not. Note that the node containing Julie's successful career has round edges to differentiate this node as a moderator. If we add these new elements to Julie's network model (and highlight the node that belongs in the dimension of motivation), it might look similar to what we can see in figure 5.3.

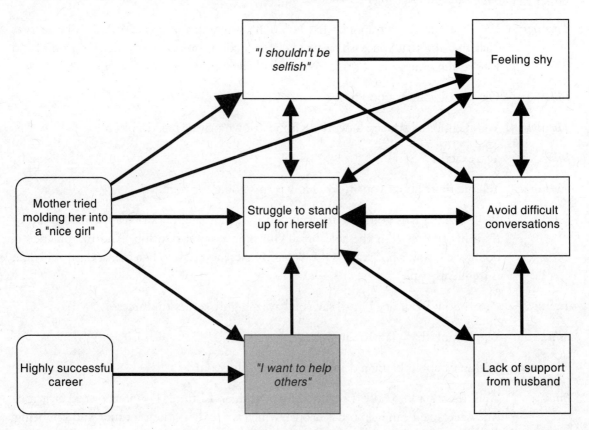

Figure 5.3 The motivational dimension

As you can see, there is predominantly one factor that belongs in the dimension of motivation, namely Julie's wish to help people other than herself. This wish is expressed in her work as a dentist (hence this relation is depicted with a simple one-way arrow), and, although some of this is a prosocial impact of her mother, that connection (her mother's influence, motivating Julie to help others) also increases her likelihood of struggling to stand up for herself.

Maladaptive motivational styles show up in many different shapes and forms. For many clients, these motivations often first present themselves in terms of what they do not want, or what they wish to avoid. However, when a therapist digs a little bit deeper, they are often able to uncover a sense of caring for something or someone. This caring can be about a specific person, about the client themself, about a group of people, about realizing a certain behavior, about achieving a certain outcome, or even about serving a cause or a beloved pet. The source of motivation can be important to guide the client to new behavior and inspire the belief that change is possible.

However, depending on the client and the function of the motivation within the network, the client's motivation might be maladaptive and actually enhance the struggle rather than soften it. This seems to be the case for Julie, as her motivation to help other people stands in seeming opposition to her ability to assert herself—at least as far as Julie's emotional reaction is concerned. She has yet to create a context in which standing up for her own needs and wishes is a clear and positive expression of caring for herself so as to care for other people. Thus, what matters more than the individual motivation is the function the motivation serves within the context of the network.

Consider the following examples of maladaptive motivation.

Material acquisition: Material acquisition refers to a motivational style whereby a person is motivated to acquire material goods, such as valuable objects. Oftentimes, the wish for material acquisition is inspired by a more deep-seated desire to feel loved, secure, and excited.

Compliance: Compliance refers to a motivational style whereby a person does not act out of their own self-interest but mindlessly adopts the values, goals, and orientations of other people around them. Oftentimes, compliance is a product of social pressure or mindless assimilation to achieve a sense of belonging with other people.

Not caring: Not caring refers to a motivational style whereby a person seemingly does not care for anything. The person acts on momentary urges and impulses rather than on higher standards or goals. Nonetheless, upon further observation, it often becomes clear that the stance of not caring is often taken to avoid feeling pain.

Naturally, there are many more examples of maladaptive motivational styles, and covering them all is, again, beyond the scope of this book. What they tend to have in common is that they speak to a surface level of caring while neglecting the underlying, more deep-seated wishes. In other words, maladaptive motivational styles speak to short-term needs and wishes, while adaptive motivational styles speak to long-term desires of the heart. Again, it is not irrational for the client to select their maladaptive motivational style. It is serving them in the short term, while being unhelpful in the long term.

As with maladaptive styles of self, instead of merely pointing out maladaptive motivations, you need to uncover the function of a specific motivational style and offer alternative strategies that access a more deep-seated sense of caring and a more flexible realization of this motivation—thus greater variation and selection. There are countless ways to do so—certainly too many to cover here—so we'll just look at a few examples of adaptive motivational styles.

Values: Values refer to inner directions toward which a person guides their actions. These inner directions have inherent worth and are not viewed by the person as a means to an end, meaning their mere pursuit is valuable in itself. The more a person lives in touch with their values, the more likely they are to take life-enhancing actions.

Goals: Goals are ideas of a desired future or future outcome that a person or a group of people envision, plan, and commit to achieve. Almost always, achieving these goals comes along with additional incentives that go beyond the goal itself.

Planning: Planning refers to envisioning and conceiving a plan of action to achieve a desired future outcome. Planning is the bridge between being motivated to take action and actually going forward and taking action.

As with the examples of maladaptive motivational styles, there are many more examples of adaptive motivational styles. At this point, it is important to (a) identify the motivational components of the client, and (b) uncover how these components fit into the client's pattern. You might find the following questions helpful in sessions with your own clients when you explore problems in variation, selection, and retention in the dimension of motivation.

Guiding Questions – Motivation

Explore problems in variation—Are there characteristic maladaptive patterns of motivation for the client when they are in their struggle, or more adaptive patterns that fail to appear that might be helpful? Is there any sense of rigidity or a lack of healthy variation in the domain of motivation?

Explore problems in selection—What are the functions of the maladaptive forms of motivation that are present in the network? When healthier forms of motivation appear, what functions might they serve?

Explore problems in retention—How do these dominant patterns in the area of motivation support, facilitate, or maintain the client's problems in the network model? In the case of more adaptive forms of motivation, why are they not retained when they occur? What other features of the network are interfering with retention of gains that may occasionally occur?

Action Step 5.2   Motivation

Considering the same problem area as before, but now focusing on motivational patterns, see if you can apply the three sets of guiding questions above to the motivation domain in your problem area. Write a paragraph about each.

Example

Problems in variation: In conversations with others, I'm primarily concerned with not embarrassing myself, or not saying something stupid. I want others to like me. I also want to be genuine and authentic, but it's so hard with my fear showing up.

Problems in selection: My motivation of "not embarrassing myself" serves to avoid getting rejected and ridiculed by others. It is a motivation primarily grounded in what I don't want, rather than what I do want. My other motivation to be genuine and authentic serves to create real connections, but it's overshadowed by my avoidance of getting hurt.

Explore problems in retention: Whenever I don't embarrass myself—which is more often than not—the belief that it didn't happen because I actively monitored myself gets reinforced. Whenever I do embarrass myself, I ascribe it to my not doing enough to avoid embarrassment. Either way, my motivation is reinforced.

THE BEHAVIORAL DIMENSION

The way clients act and behave fundamentally defines their life situation. This is true for Julie. So far into the conversation, we have uncovered several factors that show how Julie chooses to act in the middle of her struggle. For instance, Julie does not tend to stand up for herself, and even more, she tends to avoid difficult conversations entirely, thus exacerbating her struggle. However, there is more to July's story. In the subsequent conversation segment, we learn about an additional factor that shapes Julie's situation and reinforces her network.

Therapist: Let's do a quick experiment. We don't really need any equipment, and it might be insightful for you about how we can bring about change.

Julie: Okay, sure.

Therapist: Suppose I had a gun in my hand. And I would point this gun at you, and I would tell you that I will shoot unless you feel the confidence you need to stand up for yourself. And I'm talking about genuine confidence. Not fake confidence. So unless you feel really confident, I would shoot you. Now how do you think this will go?

Julie: Well, you will probably shoot me.

Therapist: Yes, exactly. I would notice you don't feel fully confident, and I would shoot you. Now suppose we do it a little differently: I would shoot you unless you genuinely believed that you have what it takes to stand up to me. And for some reason I could really tell if you are faking it. Now what would happen?

Julie: I guess I would be shot again.

Therapist: I agree. So, there's no winning here. Now let's try this one last time, but this time I would tell you that I will shoot you unless you say "No." No big explanation, and no assertive facial expressions, but just uttering the word "No." Do you think you would be able to make it?

Julie: Of course. I might want to cry, but I would say "No."

Therapist: The point of this little exercise is that it's much easier to change our actual behaviors than to change how we think and feel. And if we want to make a change, it's often best to start by looking at our behavior—the things we actually do—as a place to start. Let's look at what you are actually doing when you are struggling. So far you have mentioned that you tend to avoid difficult conversations, and that you do not speak up for yourself.

Julie: Right.

Therapist: These things are really about *not* doing something. *Not* speaking up, and *not* having a difficult conversation. And when you are in a difficult moment with someone, what do you actually *do*?

Julie: I just try to please. My husband calls me a "people pleaser." I think it actually annoys him even though he'll also do things like tell me not to go to this conference. I know when I say, "I'm going," he'll back down, but it's just hard for me emotionally, especially when I'm already feeling nervous. That's really why I'm here. I know I have to change my behavior.

In this last segment, we have learned a few more crucial things about Julie's situation. We have learned that Julie often behaves in passive ways, where she avoids conflict and difficult conversations. Instead, she resorts to people pleasing—especially when she fears disapproval from another person. If we add this new element to Julie's network model along with its relations to other factors, and highlight the factors that revolve around behavior, it might look similar to what we can see in figure 5.4.

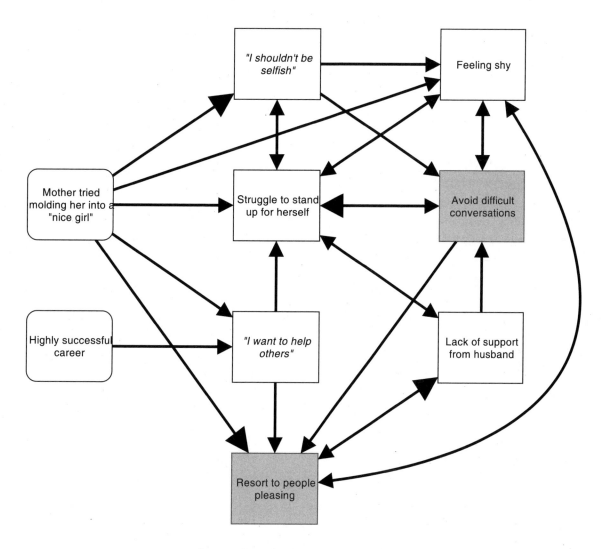

Figure 5.4 The behavioral dimension

Naturally, Julie's unwillingness to speak up for her needs and wishes and to have difficult conversations fundamentally creates difficulties in her relationships. Furthermore, her tendency to resort to people pleasing is a product of multiple factors, including her upbringing, her desire to help others, and her unwillingness to have difficult conversations (hence all of these relations are depicted with a simple one-way arrow, albeit the influence of her mother was most likely the dominant factor). Additionally, when her husband meets Julie with disapproval, she engages even more in people pleasing, while simultaneously, her people pleasing is actually putting off her husband. In other words, the nodes "Lack of support from husband" and "Resort to people pleasing" bidirectionally influence and strengthen each other (hence the relationship is depicted as a two-way arrow). Something similar happens when Julie feels shy, where her feelings of shyness lead her to resort even more to people-pleasing behavior, which in turn further fuels her fear-based feelings (i.e., if the situation were entirely "safe," she wouldn't have needed to resort to people pleasing in the first place, thus she "justifies" her feelings of shyness). As a result, this relationship too is depicted as a double-headed arrow.

A client's behavior often stands in the center of their struggle, as is true for Julie. Her struggle is maintained and facilitated by her unwillingness to speak up for her needs and engage in confrontation, while simultaneously resorting to "people pleasing." Nonetheless, these behaviors—while maladaptive and increasing long-term suffering—serve an important function for Julie. By disengaging from difficult conversations, she disengages from difficult thoughts, feelings, and other internal experiences that might occur in the moment. In other words, her passive style is a coping mechanism to help her avoid feeling uncomfortable, which is part of why she repeats the behavior.

Many maladaptive behaviors are comforting in the short term while creating costs in the long run. Note that all this reasoning about Julie's situation will be analyzed more properly within the context of a functional analysis linked to additional data. At this point, it's important to note that behaviors that increase long-term suffering often seem positive in the short term.

Consider the following examples of maladaptive behaviors.

Avoidance: Avoidance refers to a behavioral style whereby a person acts to avoid situations where they would get in contact with undesirable thoughts, feelings, and other internal experiences. Oftentimes, this avoidant behavior is pleasant in the short term (as it removes the undesirable experience) while having long-term costs for the person's goals and general well-being.

Impulsivity: Impulsivity refers to a behavioral style whereby a person acts out of momentary urges and impulses. This behavior is often pleasurable in the short term while being reckless and coming to the detriment of larger long-term goals and objectives.

Procrastination: Procrastination refers to a behavioral style whereby a person postpones acting on their goals and objectives to avoid contact with uncomfortable internal experiences such as stress, anxiety, strain, and boredom. Procrastination often consumes a lot of time and energy while postponing desired future outcomes.

Naturally, there are many more examples of maladaptive behavioral styles, and covering them all would—yet again—defeat the purpose of this book. What they all have in common is that they remove immediate discomfort in the short term while maintaining discomfort in the long term, thus reinforcing the maladaptive behavioral style and creating a loop. Again, it is not irrational for the client to select their maladaptive behavioral style. It is just not working in their favor.

As with maladaptive self-styles and motivational styles, beyond merely pointing out maladaptive behavioral styles, you need to uncover the function of a specific behavior and offer viable alternative strategies that allow broader, more flexible behavior, and thus greater variation. Again, the ways to do so are too many to mention, so instead of covering them all, let's take a look at some examples of adaptive behavioral styles.

Commitment: Commitment refers to a behavioral style whereby a person has made a promise to themself or others about engaging in a certain behavior to achieve a desired future outcome. Oftentimes this promise is accompanied with a specific plan of action, specifying when, where, and how to act, so that the person has maximum likelihood of success.

Behavioral activation: Behavioral activation refers to a behavioral style whereby a person starts by putting forward action without necessarily being motivated by internal experiences, such as thoughts, feelings, or other impulses. This therapeutic intervention is often used to treat people with depression.

Problem solving: Problem solving refers to a behavioral style whereby a person engages in an active process of finding a solution for a difficult issue presenting itself. Oftentimes, the person has a desired future outcome in mind toward which they are working.

As with the examples of maladaptive behavioral styles, there are more examples of adaptive behavioral styles. At this point in therapy, it is important to (a) identify the client's behavioral components, and (b) uncover how these components fit into the client's pattern. You might find the following questions helpful in sessions with your own clients when you explore problems in variation, selection, and retention in the dimension of behavior.

Guiding Questions – Behavior

Explore problems in variation—What patterns of overt behavior show up for the client when they are in their struggle, or fail to appear that might be helpful? Is there any sense of rigidity or a lack of healthy variation in the domain of overt behavioral patterns or habits?

Explore problems in selection—What are the functions of problematic forms of overt behavior in the client's network? If or when more adaptive forms of overt behavior appear, what functions might these overt action patterns serve?

Explore problems in retention—How do these dominant overt behavioral patterns support, facilitate, or maintain the client's problems in the network model? In the case of more adaptive overt patterns of action, why are they not retained when they occur? What other features of the network are interfering with retention of behavioral gains that may occasionally occur?

Action Step 5.3   Behavior

See if you can apply the three sets of guiding questions above to the dimension of overt behavior in the problem area of yours that you selected to work on. Write a paragraph about each.

Example

Problems in variation: When I get nervous in social situations, I either overcompensate and try to be the funniest, most interesting person in the room, or I retreat, often excusing myself and going home. It's almost always one or the other.

Problems in selection: I overcompensate in the hopes of being more liked by others and building close relationships. On the other hand, I retreat in order to not get hurt by others. I reject myself before I can get rejected by others.

Explore problems in retention: When I overcompensate and other people react positively, I assume it must have been because I put on a show. When they react negatively, however, I assume it must have been because I didn't try hard enough. Either way, the behavior is reinforced. Whenever I retreat, the nervousness and fear dissipate; thus, the behavior is reinforced.

FUNCTIONAL ANALYSIS OF JULIE

In many ways, we've already done a functional analysis of this case in the chapter. Julie's pressing issue and the larger pattern she is worried about is giving in to unreasonable demands and avoiding difficult conversations if it means standing up for herself. This pattern has a history in her family of origin, which included fairly strong parenting linked to being a "nice girl" who avoids being "selfish."

Given that history, acting in ways that serve her own interests will not only lead readily to thoughts of being selfish, but it will also make her feel as though her actions threaten her being loved or cared for. Avoiding difficult conversations about her own needs, even at the cost of her own self-respect or ability to play a role as the highly competent professional she is, feels "safe" and, superficially, seems loving. This is not all "in her head"—it is in the social contingencies Julie experiences. It's a socially supported and gender-biased narrative that began with her mother and continues with her husband. But changing those contingencies also requires behavior change on Julie's part.

Julie's core motivation is to help people, which she does professionally and personally. In the specific incident that led her to come in for therapy, her desire to go to a professional conference is blocked by her husband. The problem is that steps in the direction of helping others can call forth the thought that she is doing it "on the backs of other people," and there we are, back to people pleasing and avoiding difficult conversations—which hold the system together.

The therapist has focused on overt behavior in this last section of the case, emphasizing the idea that it can be changed more readily than habitual thoughts or feelings. However, changes in behavior will not be sustained unless they are connected to deeper motivation, which will guide the work of addressing the underlying issues of her own self narrative.

One way to perturbate this set of functional relations is to introduce variations in the relevant EEMM dimensions with the goal of selecting and retaining more adaptive alternatives. One promising approach might be to arrange for "difficult conversations" with her husband in therapy, especially if Julie could link her motivation to step forward professionally and personally with a real desire to help people. Standing up for herself is necessary for her to "be herself" and to contribute. We do not know if a genuine, open, values-based conversation with her husband will move the needle in her relationship with her husband, or her own self-narrative, but it is time to find out.

Action Step 5.4   Fill in Your EEMM:
Self, Motivational, and Behavioral Dimensions

Let's return to the problem you identified in your own life. Please draw a partial EEMM based on what you wrote in Action Steps 5.1 through 5.3, and fill in the relevant dimensions as they relate to your problem. As in chapter 4, your problem may not be very well represented in all dimensions or in all columns, so we are still not including retention and context specificity columns. Also, we are focusing here on maladaptive areas, but you can add adaptive things you could do if you wish.

	MALADAPTIVE	
	Variation	Selection
Self		
Motivation		
Behavior		

Example

	MALADAPTIVE	
	Variation	Selection
Self	I think I'm a total loser and simply not good enough. These thoughts seem very convincing.	Well, by rejecting myself first, I protect myself from getting hurt by others.
Motivation	I'm primarily concerned with not embarrassing myself, or not saying something stupid. I want others to like me. I also want to be genuine and authentic, but it's so hard with my fear showing up.	I don't want to get rejected or ridiculed. I also want to be genuine and authentic to create real connections, but it's often overshadowed.
Behavior	I either overcompensate and try to be the most interesting person in the room, or I retreat, often excusing myself and going home.	I overcompensate to be more liked by others and build close relationships. On the other hand, I retreat in order to not get hurt anymore.

CHAPTER 6

The Biophysiological and Sociocultural Levels

Michael was formerly addicted to alcohol and experiences cognitive impairments. He struggles to maintain his focus, is easily distractible, and—as of late—has become quite forgetful. He now worries that his years of drinking have finally caught up with him and left a mark.

In the previous two chapters, we explored the six dimensions of the Extended Evolutionary Meta-Model (namely cognition, affect, attention, self, motivation, and overt behavior). In this chapter, we expand our understanding of the EEMM by adding the biophysiological and sociocultural levels. These two levels set the context for the six dimensions, and both levels fundamentally influence a client's condition and overall well-being—for better or worse.

Parenthetically, you may have noticed that we are using a relatively uncommon term, *biophysiology*, for a suborganismic level of analysis. We are doing so because "physiology" is too narrow (the evolutionary history of genetics is not usually considered to be part of "physiology"), but "biological" is too vague and all-encompassing and is often used at the level of the whole organism (many psychologists would comfortably cast all of psychology as "biological," for example). The term biophysiology is rarely used in a technical way, but it has been previously used as a generic label, much in the way we are using it here to encompass a level of analysis that includes time scales that can range from milliseconds to eons.

In the following section, we will see how Michael's history of alcohol addiction continues to affect him, and we'll learn about the role played by biophysiologically relevant actions and his sociocultural background. We start with a conversation between the therapist and Michael, and accordingly organize the gathered information into a network model.

MICHAEL'S MORNING FOG

Therapist: What brings you here today?

Michael: To be up front, it wasn't my idea. My doctor recommended I come see you, because you might be able to help me.

Therapist: Why don't you start by telling me what I can do for you?

Michael: Yes, sure. Lately, I have had this morning fog more often. I cannot concentrate like I used to, I get distracted, and I'm just off. It's incredibly frustrating, and it's starting to make me worry about my performance at work.

Therapist: And what type of work do you do?

Michael: I run a paper supply company. It's growing. It's successful. I have a decent-sized staff, and most of my job is about supervising, managing resources, and making sure everything runs smoothly.

Therapist: So, it would be fair to say that you need your full focus.

Michael: Yes, that would be fair to say. And I feel like I'm not quite on my game, and I worry about what it might mean for my company.

Therapist: When you notice that you aren't as focused as you used to be, you begin to worry about your work performance.

Michael: Yeah. I mean, I've built this company from the ground up, quite successfully even. But if I can't focus, I won't be able to run it as I should. As I said, I feel incredibly frustrated by it, and then worry even more, which frustrates me even more (*chuckles*).

In the first few moments of the conversation, we have already learned important details about Michael's situation. We have learned that Michael has a "morning fog," where he loses his focus. Furthermore, we have learned that Michael is a highly successful entrepreneur, running his own paper supply company. The morning fog is an issue, and it makes Michael feel frustrated and worry about his work performance. The feelings of frustration seem to further fuel Michael's tendency to worry, which in turn again increases his feelings of frustration. When we put these elements of Michael's case (as well as their underlying relations) into a network, it might look similar to what we see in figure 6.1.

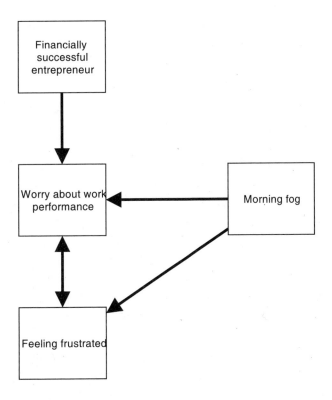

Figure 6.1 Michael's initial network model

Therapist: You mentioned that you worry a lot about your work performance. What do you exactly do when this worry shows up?

Michael: I don't think there's much to do about it. I simply have to deal with it. I'm not really here to talk about my worry; I'm here because I cannot work like I used to anymore.

Therapist: Okay, then let's talk about your work and your morning fog. What do you think might be the reason that it is showing up now?

Michael: I actually have a theory, but it scares me. A couple of years ago, I used to be a somewhat heavy drinker, drinking hard liquor almost every day. And I think it might have something to do with it.

Therapist: And how long have you been sober now?

Michael: Around five years. I started going to AA meetings, which I still attend every week. It made a big difference. But now I fear that I might have caused some irreparable damage to myself. Maybe early Alzheimer's or something.

Therapist: So, you think that your past alcohol abuse might cause your mental fog?

Michael: Yes. And I also have had some trouble sleeping lately, which I can tell is also draining me.

Therapist: Can you tell me more about your sleep problems?

Michael: I've never been much of a sleeper, like maybe six hours a night. But lately it's been more like five. I have a hard time even falling asleep.

In conversation with the therapist, Michael has revealed new important details, which we can use to expand his network model. We have learned that Michael's struggle with morning fog might be due to his history with alcohol abuse. He used to drink hard liquor daily but has been sober for five years. Nonetheless, he still attends weekly Alcoholics Anonymous meetings, as he feels they are helping him. Next, Michael experiences difficulties falling asleep and only sleeps five hours a night, which might add to his morning fog. Since quality of sleep strongly correlates with a person's ability to focus, we suspect a strong influence of "Sleep problems" on "Morning fog." Lastly, Michael reported that he needs to deal with his worry by himself. It might be that his worry reveals a failure on Michael's part to reach out for help and structure an environmental support system for self-care. At this point, this is merely a speculation. We will further investigate this assumption as we continue our work with Michael. If we add these new elements (as well as their relations) to Michael's network model, it might look similar to what we can see in figure 6.2. Please note that the node for Michael's history with alcohol addiction has round edges to differentiate it as a moderator.

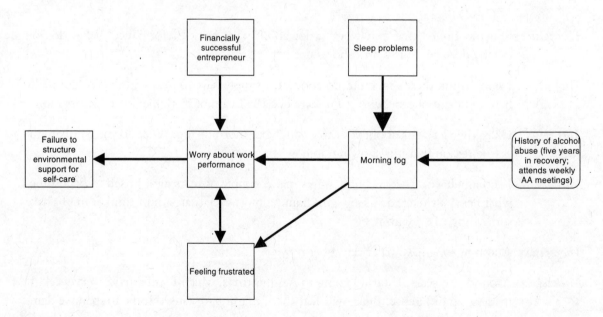

Figure 6.2 Michael's expanded network model

The factors we have just put into nodes (as well as their underlying relations) represent the core of Michael's situation. So far, the network consists of no self-reinforcing cycle involving more than two nodes. As we continue the conversation between the therapist and Michael, we explore the biophysiological and sociocultural levels and uncover additional elements and relations to further make sense of Michael's situation and identify sensitive nodes that would lend themselves to be disrupted through interventions.

THE BIOPHYSIOLOGICAL LEVEL

What we call "the body" and what we call "the mind" are two levels of the same system—they are fundamentally interconnected, and you cannot treat one without affecting the other. This is the starting point of the biophysiological level of the EEMM, where we explore the client's biology, how they treat their own body, and how their physiology affects their overall well-being. Naturally, genetic differences always play a big role in determining a client's vulnerabilities and strengths. And through epigenetic markers, gene expression is influenced. In some areas, parents and grandparents can affect a client through their behavioral choices and experiences, even those that occurred before the client was born. In some way, for example, a client's food preferences may be the result of a grandfather's eating habits above and beyond the issue of family traditions and culture.

Biological differences play a notable role in shaping the client's life. As the role of epigenetics and brain circuits becomes more known and modifiable, this level of analysis will become more practically important. But, at the present time, when it comes to biophysiological interventions, therapists almost always put the focus on the same three areas: diet, exercise, and sleep.

All three of these areas fundamentally influence a person's biological well-being. And if any of these areas is off (let alone all of these areas), the client will feel the effects almost immediately. Additionally, the client's lifestyle choices can play a big role in shaping their physical well-being—for better or worse. Practices like regular meditation and taking cold showers might increase a client's well-being, whereas excessive sitting or smoking tends to deteriorate it. In short, there are a lot of factors for therapists to take into account when exploring the biophysiological level. So, let's see what this might look like in session, when the therapist explores these features of the biophysiological level together with Michael.

Therapist: It's not exactly a secret, but however we treat our bodies shapes how we think and feel about ourselves.

Michael: Yes? And so?

Therapist: If you don't mind, I'd like to explore a little bit about how you are treating your own body, because I think it might give us valuable insights about your morning fog and struggle to focus. Is this okay?

Michael: Yes. Sure. As you can see, I have a bit of a belly. I gained some pounds when I was drinking, and I've never been able to shake it off.

Therapist: I think it might play a role in your struggle. And you know, when it comes to taking care of our bodies, it's always the same three things that matter: sleep, diet, and exercise. We have already talked about your sleep, so we can skip this. But how do you feel about your diet? What do you eat on a normal day?

Michael: It depends really. I know I don't eat lots of greens like I'm supposed to. I got a lot of things on my mind, and eating healthy is not exactly one of them. I eat a lot of takeout, especially when I stress about work.

Therapist: And what kind of takeout are we talking about?

Michael: I love Southern food and really any kind of meat. That's what my family ate—so that's what I know to cook when I'm home. But even when I'm out eating other kinds of food, fat and meat just draw me in. There's this Italian place I really like—there it's pizza with pepperoni—and there's a great Chinese place, but there it's fried duck.

Therapist: Got it. And what do you normally drink when you order?

Michael: Coke, mostly. Or any kind of soda. I really got into that when I stopped with the hard stuff. I feel like it really helped me through that period. They say alcohol is similar to sugar, and I get a kind of sugar craving that I satisfy with soda. That's been true ever since I was sober.

Therapist: And where does exercise fall in here? Do you exercise?

Michael: No, not really. I used to when I was in my twenties, but with the job and everything, I feel like I have no time for it. And in a way, the belly makes it even harder to get going. I know, I just gotta start somewhere.

Therapist: What do you think needs to happen so you can start again?

Michael: Nothing really. I just got to start doing it. I don't like these yuppie weight loss programs. You know, I think you should be able to do it yourself. That's how things were in my family: just do it. I just have to get started.

Therapist: So you haven't been sleeping very well, you eat lots of takeout, and you don't exercise. It might very well be that all of these have been affecting you more than you might think. When was your last physical checkup? Do you have any physical complaints?

Michael: Yes…not too long ago. My doctor was the one who actually recommended that I come to see you. I've been dealing with hypertension, and, well, my belly has grown as I already said. My father is a diabetic, and my doctor was worried that I was moving in a similar direction.

Through this last conversation segment, we have gathered new puzzle pieces, which we can now add to Michael's network model to further inform his case. First, we have learned that Michael has been overweight for the last several years, and that this might be due to his not eating well and not exercising. Additionally, it might be a relic of his history with alcohol abuse that he hasn't yet been able to shake off. His "Southern cooking" food preference is fatty meat, and he eats a lot of take-out food, especially when stressed about work, mostly sticking with fatty meat or sugary sodas. His poor sleep might also contribute to his eating habits, and his poor diet in turn might contribute to his sleeping problems (hence the relation in figure 6.3 is depicted as a double-headed arrow).

Michael does not believe that group programs might be able to help him lose weight or exercise more, and instead is convinced that this is something he "should be able to do by [himself]." This might be yet another indicator that he fails to build an environmental support system for self-care (which may sound ironic, given his positive experience with AA meetings, which he still attends to this day). Nonetheless, his belief of having to do things "yourself" might have brought him to become a financially successful entrepreneur, and his success might have only further reinforced his do-it-yourself attitude.

Michael might experience more morning fog because he does not exercise. And because he experiences morning fog, he might struggle to exercise in the first place (which is why this relation is also depicted as a double-headed arrow). The same seems true for his weight, where Michael's body weight makes it harder for him to get started exercising. It is also noteworthy that his lack of exercise likely contributes directly to his sleeping problems. Lastly, Michael reported that he has hypertension, which might be a direct result of his body weight, eating habits, lack of exercise, and history with alcohol abuse.

Subsequently, we now add these new elements (as well as their interconnected relations) to Michael's network model. If we highlight those nodes that belong to the biophysiological level, it might look similar to what we can see in figure 6.3.

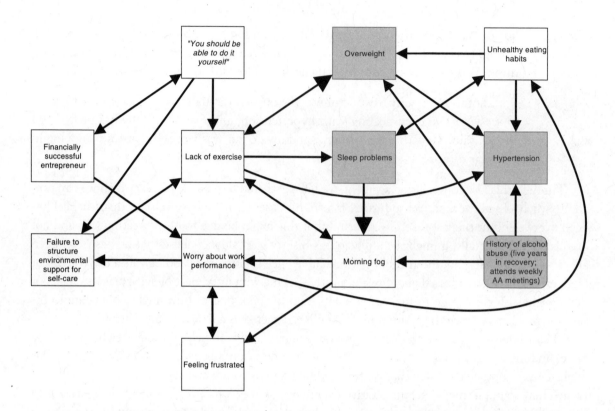

Figure 6.3 The biophysiological level

As you can see, Michael's network model has become much more complex and detailed, giving us new insights into his condition and what maintains and facilitates his struggle. It becomes apparent that Michael is neglectful of his physical health and fails to attend to his self-care. As a result, he experiences difficulties sleeping, has become overweight, and experiences hypertension, which ultimately all likely contribute to Michael's morning fog.

Now that the network model has become more complex, we can identify several self-reinforcing network loops. In the most central loop, Michael's morning fog reinforces his worry about work, which in turn reinforces processes that lead him to neglect his self-care, which exacerbate his sleep problems and subsequently his morning fog. Furthermore, there is a self-reinforcing cycle between "Lack of exercise" and "Overweight," where a lack of exercise contributes to Michael's being overweight and vice versa. Similarly, there are self-reinforcing loops between other pairs of factors, such as "Lack of exercise" and "Morning fog," "Sleep problems" and "Unhealthy eating habits," and "Financially successful entrepreneur" and the belief that "You should be able to do it yourself."

Another more complex self-sustaining subnetwork stems from Michael's morning fog, which makes it harder for him to exercise, thus exacerbating his sleep problems, which reinforces his morning fog again. And lastly, there is a subnetwork stemming from Michael's lack of exercise, which exacerbates his sleep problems, leading to unhealthy eating, which contributes to Michael's being overweight, which also makes it harder for him to exercise.

The network model of Michael is not yet complete, and we will expand it in later sections of the chapter when we explore the role of the sociocultural level. For now, it's important to note the effect his biophysiological level has on his well-being, which is profound. His difficulty with morning fog (as well as other related problems) is directly maintained and exacerbated by factors concerning his physical health. As a result, Michael would be well advised to attend to his physical self-care in order to improve his morning clarity and concentration. Furthermore, it would be of interest for the therapist to further explore and identify factors and obstacles that stand in the way of Michael's taking steps to improve his physical health. Again, all elements will be analyzed more deeply in a functional analysis in a later part of the chapter.

The state of the biophysiological level of a client profoundly affects and influences their mental well-being. Specifically, the following three areas are highly important:

Diet: "You are what you eat" is not only a common saying, it's also true. The quality of food we consume (as well as the quantity) fundamentally influences not only our weight but our overall health, and thus all processes concerning our mental health. Especially in the US, the average diet consistently contains too much sugar and salt and too few healthy nutrients.

Exercise: The benefit of regular exercise to our physical and mental well-being has been well documented. Those who fail to regularly move their body can expect to suffer the consequences as their bodies become heavy, inflexible, and stiff with age. And even in the short term, a person's level of exercise has a big effect on their physical and mental well-being.

Sleep: We need our sleep in order to function. The amount of sleep each of us requires may differ, but there is little doubt about the importance of sleep for our physical and mental health. Whether a client gets enough sleep, as well as the quality of their sleep, may be an important factor that can improve or worsen a client's condition.

Naturally, there are many more relevant areas to explore within the biophysiological level. For instance, a client's activities throughout the day (e.g., excessive sitting, smoking, meditation) can fundamentally affect their physical health beyond the previously mentioned factors. It is not the aim of this volume to give a detailed description about the many ways in which clients help or harm their physical well-being. Instead, we want to point out the role that the biophysiological level plays in initiating, maintaining, and exacerbating a client's condition.

It does not suffice to merely point out ways in which clients contribute to their poor physical health, just as it does not suffice to merely point out that smoking causes cancer to convince a smoker to stop. Instead, you will need to identify the function of a specific behavior (or lack thereof) and help the client build effective, alternative strategies that allow for more flexible behavior in line with the client's biophysiological goals.

At this point in therapy, it is important to (a) identify the client's components related to the biophysiological level, and (b) uncover how these components fit into the client's overall pattern.

You might find the following guiding questions helpful in sessions with your own clients when you explore problems in your client's biophysiological level.

Guiding Questions – Biophysiological Level

Explore problems in variation—What biophysiologically relevant behavior patterns show up for the client when they are in their struggle, or fail to appear that might be helpful? Is there any sense of rigidity or a lack of healthy variation in the level of these biophysiologically relevant actions (e.g., failure to try healthier eating, unwillingness to explore ways to exercise)?

Explore problems in selection—What are the functions of problematic biophysiologically relevant actions in the client's network? For example, does not exercising allow them to avoid experiencing shame about their body? Are poor eating patterns cultural? If or when more adaptive forms of the biophysiological level appear, what functions might these patterns serve?

Explore problems in retention—How do these dominant biophysiologically relevant patterns support, facilitate, or maintain the client's problems in the network model? In the case of more adaptive biophysiological patterns, why are they not retained when they occur? What other features of the network are interfering with retention of biophysiologically relevant gains that may occasionally occur?

In order to explore these key questions, you will also need to know a lot about key biophysiologically relevant actions. These questions are more of the common sense type, but they include:

Explore adaptive and maladaptive patterns in diet

- What do you eat that is healthy/unhealthy in an average day?

- How often and when do you overeat, or restrict what you eat?

- What do you drink? And how much?

Explore adaptive and maladaptive patterns in exercise

- Do you exercise? How often?

- What type of exercise do you do?

- How intensely do you exercise?

- How long have you been exercising/not been exercising?

Explore problems in sleep

- How well do you sleep?
- Do you experience difficulty falling asleep?
- What time do you go to sleep/wake up?
- Do you feel rested after sleeping?

Explore problems in other health-related habits

- Do you take any drugs? If so, what, how often, and how much?
- How much time in a day do you spend sitting?
- Do you meditate? If so, how often and for how long?
- How much time do you spend outside?
- How do you relax?

Action Step 6.1   Biophysiological Level

Let's return to the problem area you identified in your own life. Consider the three sets of guiding questions above and answer each related to selection, variation, and retention. Do the answers appear to be of relevance to your problem? If so, write about how these areas may restrict or foster healthy variation and the selection or retention of gains.

Example

Problems in variation: When I get scared, I notice my stomach tightening. Everything in me feels like it's getting pulled together. My heart beats faster, I tend to sweat more, and I notice that I get fidgety.

Problems in selection: I assume it's my body's way of preparing myself for danger. My body wants to protect me, but it actually makes it harder for me.

Problems in retention: When my fear gets to be too much, I just leave. I almost always let my fear control me, and therefore the fear and the biophysiological symptoms remain (or even grow stronger). In my struggle, I'm much too agitated to calm down and relax.

THE SOCIOCULTURAL LEVEL

The family and culture we grow up in has a lasting effect on how we view and treat ourselves and the challenges we encounter in our lifetime. And even when we separate from our family and culture, our social network (e.g., friends, neighbors, colleagues) and new culture we choose to live in continue to affect our mental well-being. This is the reason why any conversation about mental health is not complete until we talk about the sociocultural level.

In this part of the EEMM, we consider the social context of a client and how the client gives meaning to their struggle and their path to betterment through their social and cultural beliefs. Naturally, different cultures are differently accepting of difficult thoughts, emotions, and other internal experiences—especially when those experiences touch on topics of sexuality, morality, ethnic identity, and social status. As a result, the client's mental state may move in a more compassionate, flexible direction, or in a direction of judgment and rigidity.

In addition to the client's cultural beliefs (and those of their social network), it is important to investigate the level of social support the client experiences. Even within a particular culture, the level of social support differs widely among individuals, and it is yet another crucial factor that shapes a person's ability to cope with difficult experiences.

In the following conversation piece, the therapist will explore the sociocultural context that has made Michael who he is, and how his identity as an African American man has shaped his well-being.

Therapist: We have talked a bit about how your body affects your well-being, but there are also other factors that might play an important role, like your thoughts and beliefs. And if you're willing, I'd like to use our remaining time to highlight a bit of those other factors.

Michael: I'm listening.

Therapist: You mentioned that group exercise or weight loss programs are not for you. And in order to lose weight, you "just have to get started." And even earlier, you mentioned that your worry is something you have to "deal with yourself." It sounds as though you are very used to solving your own problems.

Michael: Well, yeah. That's how it works. No one else is going to do it for me.

Therapist: Understood. And it seems this approach has been working well for you at work, where you managed to build your own business. Have you always had to fix your problems by yourself? Is this how problems were solved in your family?

Michael: Yes, I think so. My parents aren't rich. Me and my sisters grew up in a poor household, and both my dad and mom had to take on multiple jobs just to keep the lights on.

They aren't the most educated folks, but they always had a lift-yourself-up mentality. I think it really made an impression on me.

Therapist: It is quite common for people to adopt the work mentality of their parents. Your life history shows how a "do-it-yourself" attitude can be helpful when it comes to building a business, for instance, but it can also complicate things when it comes to, let's say, self-care, because some things are easier done with social or professional support.

Michael: Well, that's true. I still think it's unnecessary. These overpriced programs are pretty pretentious. I don't have to go to a jogging group to know how to walk. I know how to use my legs.

Therapist: That's an interesting way of putting it. Is this something you learned from your family as well?

Michael: Probably, yes. My family didn't really have much, and in my dad's generation being pretentious or acting as if you are better pretty much guaranteed you a beating. At least that's what my dad always said. I mean, I've never witnessed it, but my dad did.

Therapist: May I ask how your family talked about prejudice?

Michael: My family was never big on talking about difficult subjects. They just urged me to be hard working...and taught me to like greasy food! (laughs). In all seriousness, they taught me to keep my head down and keep focused, but they are not exactly open-minded. They don't know that I'm gay, for instance. I don't think they would under-stand. They don't really understand many things about my life, because they are still set in their old ways. It's okay. I see the folks at AA more like my family anyway.

The last conversation segment provided us with new puzzle pieces to further build out Michael's network model. For instance, we learned that Michael's identity as a gay African American man has shaped his relationship with his family as well as his social values. Since Michael's ethnic and sexual identity as well as his family and social values are moderators, we put these factors in nodes with round edges. Michael seems to have two central beliefs that could explain and maintain his rigid behavior. First, he seems to believe that he should be able to do things by himself. This do-it-yourself attitude has helped Michael to become a financially successful entrepreneur, but it might also stand in the way of his building a support structure for his self-care and prevent him from joining a workout group or a weight loss program. Second, Michael seems to hold firm to the belief that "you shouldn't act like you are better." While seemingly humble on the surface, this belief might prevent him yet again from attending support groups that could help him exercise more and lose weight. These two beliefs seem to be related and feed into each other, since Michael seems to have made a connection where "not acting like you are better" means "doing things by yourself" (which is why the relationship is depicted as a double-headed arrow in figure 6.4). Lastly, Michael mentioned in an off-note that his family taught him to like "greasy food," which most likely influenced his unhealthy eating habits. If we add those new elements to Michael's network model (and highlight those nodes that belong to the sociocultural level), it might look similar to what we can see in figure 6.4.

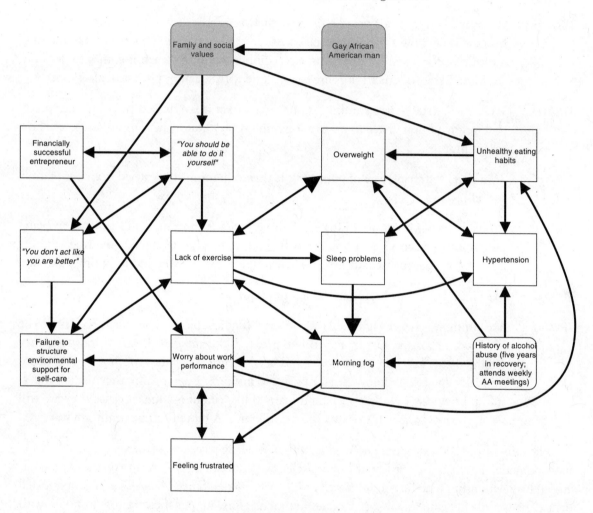

Figure 6.4 The sociocultural level

As you can see, Michael's network model has reached a new level of complexity, and it gives us new insights into his condition and what maintains and facilitates his struggle. It becomes clear that Michael has two central beliefs that have aided him in life (i.e., enabled him to become a successful entrepreneur) but that also have hindered him from seeking out and accepting help. Again, this may sound contradictory, given his previous positive experience with AA meetings, from which he continues to draw support. He may yet need to see how his family's belief system is now posing a challenge for him and that he may need to replace old-fashioned values with new, more flexible, and more adaptive beliefs that will help him better reach his goals. Even though there are no new self-sustaining network loops, the sociocultural level gives new meaning to Michael's behavior. Furthermore, by disrupting his beliefs "You don't act like you are better" and "You should be able to do it yourself," it might be possible to disrupt neighboring processes that would enable him to build a support structure for self-care.

When, where, and how Michael's network is best disrupted will be discussed in a later section when we make a functional analysis of Michael's case. At this point, it's important to note the effect his sociocultural level has on his mental well-being and overall network. His upbringing and cultural beliefs have a direct effect on his failure to build a support structure for self-care, which in turn maintains factors that contribute to Michael's morning fog. As a result, Michael would be well advised to challenge some of these family and cultural values to help him build a better support structure for self-care and thus improve his chances at betterment.

The sociocultural level of a client provides the context for the six dimensions of the EEMM and gives meaning to the client's situation. Oftentimes it circles back to these three areas:

Cultural beliefs: Cultural beliefs are like air. You cannot see them, but they constantly surround you. The beliefs a client has about themselves and their environment fundamentally shape their condition, especially when those beliefs touch on topics of sexuality, morality, ethnic identity, and social status.

Social support: The degree to which a person experiences social support fundamentally shapes their ability to cope with difficult experiences. A person with a rich social network, filled with supportive friends and family members, will be better able to bounce back from adversity than a person with poor social support.

Stigma: The prejudice and stigma a person is exposed to can heavily wear on their mental well-being. This is especially true if the person is part of a disenfranchised group (and even more so when they are part of more than one such group, like a gay African American man).

Naturally, there are many more relevant areas within the sociocultural level that are worth exploring, like cultural traditions and social norms. Again, it is not the aim of this volume to give a detailed description about the many ways in which a client's social or cultural belonging affects their mental well-being. Instead, we want to point out the importance of the sociocultural level in initiating, maintaining, and exacerbating a client's condition. Naturally, plenty of sociocultural beliefs and behaviors overlap with a client's own beliefs and behaviors, and it is up to you to help identify maladaptive patterns and encourage the client to transform them into adaptive patterns that are in line with the client's goals.

At this point in therapy, it is important to (a) identify the client's components related to the sociocultural level, and (b) uncover how these components fit into the client's pattern. You might find the following guiding questions helpful in sessions with your own clients when you explore problems in the status of a client's sociocultural level.

Guiding Questions – Sociocultural Level

Explore problems in variation—What sociocultural patterns show up for the client when they are in their struggle, or fail to appear that might be helpful? Is there any sense of rigidity or a lack of healthy variation in the sociocultural level?

Explore problems in selection—What are the functions of problematic sociocultural patterns in the client's network? If or when more adaptive forms of the sociocultural level appear, what functions might these patterns serve?

Explore problems in retention—How do these dominant sociocultural patterns support, facilitate, or maintain the client's problems in the network model? In the case of more adaptive sociocultural patterns, why are they not retained when they occur? What other features of the network are interfering with retention of sociocultural gains that may occasionally occur?

    In order to explore these key questions, you will also need to know a lot about key socially and culturally relevant actions. These questions are more of the common sense type, but they include:

Explore issues in cultural beliefs

- What is your cultural background?
- What are your religious beliefs?
- How does your culture think about (insert critical topic of relevance to the network)?
- How are problems such as these discussed with your family and friends?
- Do you feel as though you are violating cultural norms or that you would need to do so in order to address this problem area?

Explore problems in social support

- How would you describe the relationship with your family and friends?
- How openly can you be yourself with your family and friends?
- How many close friends do you have?
- Whom do you reach out to for personal problems?

Explore problems in stigma

- What was your experience with prejudice?
- Have you been on the receiving end of prejudice?
- In which ways have you been stigmatized?
- How did prejudice affect you personally?

Action Step 6.2   Sociocultural Level

Let's return to the problem area you identified in your own life. Consider the three sets of guiding questions above and answer each. Do the answers appear to be of relevance to your problem? If so, write about how these areas may restrict or foster healthy variation and the selection or retention of gains.

Example

Problems in variation: Ever since high school, I have believed that there are "winners" and "losers." And if you're not one of the popular kids, you're a loser. If I want to be a winner, I have to be confident and charming and witty.

Problems in selection: If I explain the world to myself in these simple black/white terms, it gives me a false sense of security, because even though I end up being a loser, at least I know where I belong. Also, it gives me a strategy to feel better about myself: be more confident and more charming.

Problems in retention: The belief that there are "winners and losers" gets reinforced whenever I act on it (either by overcompensating to be a winner or by retreating to avoid feeling even more like a loser). The paradigm keeps itself in place.

FUNCTIONAL ANALYSIS OF MICHAEL

Michael's presenting problems are related to his health. He is overweight, does not exercise, has unhealthy eating habits, has hypertension, and struggles with sleep problems, which presumably give him a morning fog, contributing to his worries about his work performance. He has had alcohol abuse problems in the past, which contributes to some of these current problems. These health problems form a strong, self-sustaining network that is difficult to change (especially for the long term) through simple behavioral strategies without also addressing the core underlying issues. What are some of these core underling issues?

Upon further inquiry, it becomes clear that his health problems are closely tied to the sociocultural dimension of the EEMM. Michael's identity is as a gay African American man, and he has strong social and family values that emphasize "doing it yourself" and "not acting like you are better." This has given him a strong sense of autonomy and self-sufficiency that has served him very well in many domains of his life. For example, it helped him become a financially successful entrepreneur. But that same emphasis has made it harder to deal with worries about work performance in a healthy way and holds him back from building the necessary self-care and social support to take charge of his exercise and health goals. He has turned to unhealthy eating (which was also encouraged by family traditions), fostering sleep problems and exacerbating his morning fog, which only increases his work performance worries. Meanwhile, his unwillingness to structure environmental support for self-care inhibits him from taking more direct actions to support his health. Michael's mindset has led to a cognitively and behaviorally inflexible approach, but at the same time some of these same cognitive patterns have supported him in his work success.

If we think about this in terms of the EEMM, the rows that seem more dominant are cognition, affect, sense of self, over behavior, biophysiological patterns, and sociocultural patterns. Because we've not yet dealt with retention and context issues, we can fill out a limited EEMM for Michael.

Table 6.1 Michael's Extended Evolutionary Meta-Model

	Variation	Selection
Affect	Avoids awkward feelings about self-care.	Feels less vulnerable.
Cognition	Cognitively inflexible adoption of "do it yourself" and "don't be pretentious."	Success at business supports these patterns to a degree, as does his self-concept and his family's support of these beliefs.
Attention	Worry.	Feels functional short term but isn't in the long term.
Self	Strong identity as a gay African American man (although not out with family). Self-identity seems to restrict behavioral options, however. Self-care is something "yuppies" do.	Position of pride in family and community, and avoidance of discomfort over self-care.

Motivation	Motivated to succeed, but motivation toward self-care is restricted by cognition, sense of self, and culture.	Success at business supports these patterns.
Overt Behavior	Self-sufficient. Proven ability to run a business. Hard time engaging in self-care.	Financial and social success. Also prevents others from viewing him as self-focused.
Biophysiological	Diet, exercise, and sleep problems. "Morning fog" perhaps linked to prior drinking.	Enjoys fatty food. Motivation toward self-care buried under fused beliefs.
Sociocultural	"Do it yourself" and "don't be pretentious" are strongly inculcated. Societally, these link to history of racial prejudice. Fatty food choices are familial as well.	Positive connection to family and culture.

It becomes clear that the underlying EEMM dimensions that factor prominently in Michael's network are determined by his sociocultural background and are in turn linked to strong beliefs about autonomy and self-sufficiency. The negative consequences of these convictions are unhealthy habits leading to physical problems. Intervention strategies will need to somehow work around or modify his rigid beliefs to target the behavioral inflexibility, combined with developing motivational strategies to acquire and retain adaptive habits.

We will return to Michael's situation in chapter 9, after we assemble more features needed to begin to disrupt this system.

Action Step 6.3   Fill in Your EEMM:
Biophysiological and Sociocultural Levels

Let's return to the problem you identified in your own life. Based on your responses in Action Steps 6.1 and 6.2, fill in the partial EEMM below as it relates to your problem. Your problem may not be represented at these biophysiological or sociocultural levels. If that's the case, you can leave the relevant columns empty.

	MALADAPTIVE	
	Variation	Selection
Biophysiological		
Sociocultural		

Example

| | MALADAPTIVE | |
	Variation	Selection
Biophysiological	When I get scared, I notice my stomach tightening. Everything in me feels like it's getting pulled together. My heart beats faster, I tend to sweat more, and I notice that I get fidgety.	I assume it's my body's way of preparing myself for danger. My body wants to protect me, but actually it makes it harder for me.
Sociocultural	Ever since high school, I have believed that there are "winners" and "losers." And if you're not one of the popular kids, you're a loser. If I want to be a winner, I have to be confident and charming and witty.	Clinging to these black/white terms gives me a false sense of security, because even though I end up being a loser, at least I know where I belong. Also, it gives me a solution to feel better: be more confident and more charming.

Action Step 6.4 Create a Preliminary New Network Model

Let's return to the problem area you identified. Review your answers to the action step exercises in chapters 2 through 6. Draw a new network of events that seem to characterize it. This is similar to your task in Action Step 2.1, where you created your first network model, except now we have explored all of the dimensions and levels of the EEMM (but not yet all of the columns). Include all the relevant factors as they present themselves for you across dimensions and levels. Use as many single- or double-headed arrows as you deem necessary.

Next, write a short paragraph about what thoughts and feelings come up for you when considering this problem area from the vantage point of a more elaborate network model. Where does your mind go? How do you react when you look at this problem through the lens of this network?

Example

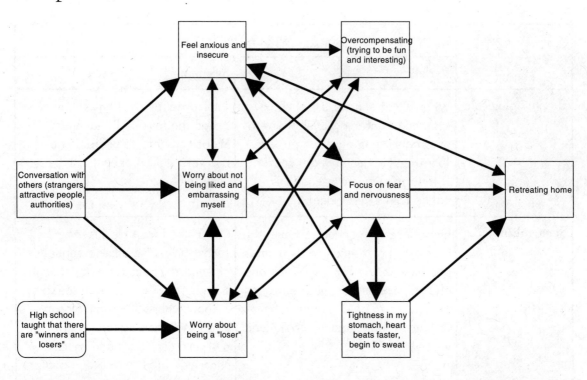

What Thoughts and Feelings Come Up for Me: I feel like I get a much better sense of everything that happens for me. I wasn't even aware of half of it. It's a lot, but also a relief, because I feel like I can get a grip on this mess. I didn't realize how important my focus on my own fear and nervousness is, and how all these elements reinforce one another. It's a big knot, but I can finally see the threads to untie it.

CHAPTER 7

Context Sensitivity and Retention

Our work as therapists is not complete until we have helped our client make an adaptive change that lasts. Before this can happen, we need to learn about the client's situation and identify the factors that maintain and exacerbate the problems. And once this has been done, we can focus on the real work: helping the client make a change by disrupting maladaptive patterns and building responses that are adaptive inside the relevant contexts.

A *context* refers to the inner and outer circumstances of the client: their personal history, genetic predisposition, cultural identity, work environment, living situation, socioeconomic status, and any other relevant setting factor that determines whether a response is adaptive or maladaptive. What may be adaptive in one context can be maladaptive in another. For instance, boasting about your achievements may land well among your friends but land poorly among your coworkers. In therapy, we aim to increase a client's context sensitivity so they become more sensitive to the demands of their context and can then flexibly adjust their response. A person who is context sensitive, for instance, knows when it's appropriate to talk openly and when it's better to keep it private.

In addition to increasing a client's context sensitivity—thus helping them choose more adaptive responses—we also want to make sure that the new response is going to stick. After all, a change is not worth much if it doesn't last beyond the therapy session. The process of solidifying new responses into full-grown habits is called *retention*. In summary, we want to help the client make a change by increasing their context sensitivity (thus strengthening their ability to notice the shifting demands of their context and choose adaptive responses) and by increasing their retention (thus strengthening their ability to make new responses stick).

For this purpose, let's revisit Maya. As you might remember, Maya had an accident at work that left her with chronic back pain. She overly focuses on her pain and frequently worries that it may never go away or that she might reinjure herself. As a result, she avoids going to work and restricts almost all of her activities. Maya thinks "it's unfair" and that her accident "shouldn't have happened" because she had previously warned her superiors about the safety hazard—but to no avail. All of her earlier complaints and warnings were noted, but not acted upon. Naturally, Maya feels a strong sense of anger over her situation, which is only growing larger. In figure 7.1. you can see the network model of Maya.

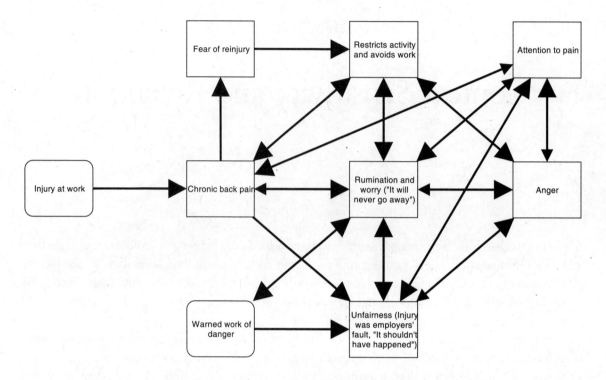

Figure 7.1. Revisiting Maya's network model

Central to Maya's struggle are her self-restriction and avoidance of work as well as her anger. Since Maya primarily sought treatment because of the latter, it would make sense to start treatment by first addressing Maya's anger. As you can see in figure 7.1, her anger is maintained and exacerbated by a number of neighboring factors revolving around her self-restriction, rumination, sense of unfairness, and excessive attention to her pain. The therapist could work on decreasing Maya's anger either directly, by adding and/or removing elements to ease her anger, or indirectly, by adding and/or removing elements that decrease the strength and influence of those neighboring factors that feed into her anger.

Once Maya's anger has lessened, it may become easier to introduce new elements to address Maya's second struggle: her tendency to restrict herself and avoid going to work. In other words, by easing her anger, the therapist might be able to get Maya to a point where she actively engages with her life once again. Before we can get there, however, we first need to address Maya's anger. As became clear from Maya's network model, one of the factors that feeds into her anger is her tendency to focus on her pain. Our first step will thus be making Maya more aware of the role of her attention within her network and how it adds to her anger. Additionally, we want to provide Maya with an alternative response, so instead of letting her attention be automatically pulled toward her pain, she can orient her focus in a more flexible, adaptive way that actually benefits her. In other words, we want to increase Maya's sensitivity to her context to enable a more flexible, adaptive response.

HOW TO INCREASE CONTEXT SENSITIVITY

Increasing a client's context sensitivity means making them more aware of the shifting demands of their context so they can flexibly adjust their response to it in an adaptive way. In order to do so, you first need to have an understanding of the client's complex situation. By being aware of the client's context, you can better understand the forces that give rise to the client's response, and thus help the client do the same. This first step—identifying central factors and determining their role within the client's problems—was done in the initial assessment phase. Once the key forces have been uncovered and the client has become aware of the demands of their context, they can actively choose alternative adaptive responses instead.

In Maya's case, there are numerous maladaptive responses that ultimately add to her anger. As we have seen, one of Maya's responses was her tendency to focus on her pain in a rigid, judgmental way. Subsequently, we must ask, which context gives rise to her response? In Maya's network model (figure 7.1), we can see that her chronic back pain, her overall sense of anger, and her sense of unfairness commonly lead Maya to focus rigidly on her pain. The therapist can then educate Maya that her focus on her pain exacerbates her anger and point out why she is likely to focus on her pain in a rigid way in the first place.

Thus, in order to increase a client's context sensitivity, you have to (1) identify the key responses within the client's network, and (2) identify the factors that reinforce and maintain those key responses. By becoming aware of the contextual demands and shifting dynamics, the client can choose alternative adaptive responses. Sometimes it's possible to change important elements within a client's context, thus making a transition to adaptive responses much easier. This is possible, for instance, when the client can remove a dysfunctional relationship that reinforces their drug habit. More often than not, however, changing important elements in the client's context is not easily done, and change needs to start with changed responses from the client. In this case, you help the client by exploring alternative responses to their contextual demands.

In Maya's case, we cannot easily get rid of her chronic back pain. Nor can we just switch off her felt anger. And although, with enough time, Maya can learn to let go of her sense of unfairness, it's more effective to start by teaching her an alternative response. Instead of focusing on her pain in a judgmental, rigid way, Maya can learn to orient her attention in a mindful, compassionate way that allows her to acknowledge her pain without getting caught up in it and paradoxically increasing its impact. Additionally, it would enable her to become more in tune with her body and explore her full range of capabilities rather than just mindlessly accepting the limitations set by her own mind. Let's see what this would look like in a therapy session.

MAYA'S MEDITATION EXERCISE

Therapist: If it's okay, I would like to do a little closed-eyes exercise with you.

Maya: You mean like a meditation?

Therapist: Something similar, yes. It's kind of guided imagery just to see how attention works in your case.

Maya: Okay, sure.

Therapist: Now, I want you to sit comfortably in your chair. And now I want you to bring awareness to the body breathing in and out. Nice and slow. In and out again. And when you're ready, intentionally breathe in, and move your attention to your body. Notice where your body touches the seat, and how the pressure feels. Notice which areas are warm, and which are cold. Which areas of your body are covered, and which are exposed. Sometimes you might notice your awareness slipping off. That's okay. Actually, it's impossible not to have that happen every now and then. Just notice that your attention has wandered off, and gently bring it back to your body. And now notice any tightness in your body. If it's possible to release it, feel free to do so. And if you can't, notice what the tightness feels like. Where it begins, and where it ends. Like a curious scientist, we just want to observe what we can notice without putting any judgment on it. And now let's move to the really painful areas. Where is your pain? What shape does it have? And what does it feel like? Don't answer these questions with words, but see if you can feel and breathe into your pain without any judgment. Just observing. Your pain is here right now, and so are you. And now move your attention to your feet. Can you sense your toes? And what about your ankles? Move your attention up your legs to your pelvis. Can you feel your belly as it moves up and down as you breathe in and out? And now move your focus even farther up to your chest. Up your arms. Can you feel your hands? And how about each finger? And now up your neck. Notice tightness in your jaw and release it. Without moving, can you feel your lips? Your ears? Your nose? Your cheeks or your forehead? And now see if you can focus your awareness on your whole body at once. And now take another deep breath in and out. And then slowly open your eyes. Welcome back!

Maya: Hello.

Therapist: Tell me, what was this like for you?

Maya: New. I never did any sort of meditation before.

Therapist:	I see. And what did you notice in your body?
Maya:	I noticed I was getting calmer. Breathing felt easier.
Therapist:	Yes, that often happens for people who meditate. And what was it like to exercise your attention in this way?
Maya:	I have to admit, I often got distracted. You were saying something one second, and I suddenly had to think about something completely different.
Therapist:	Yes, that too often happens for people who meditate. And what was it like to focus on individual body parts?
Maya:	Strange. I mean I've felt them before, but never like this. It was interesting to feel without touching it. Like a new sensation.
Therapist:	Very good. And we also talked about your pain. You mentioned that you pay a lot of attention to your pain, but I would guess that it's different from the way we just did it in the exercise, is this right?
Maya:	Yeah. I mean, when I focus on my pain it just becomes bigger and bigger, and just consumes me. And how we did it just now felt a bit lighter. I mean, it's still there, it still hurts.
Therapist:	Yes, and unfortunately, no form of meditation will completely take your pain away. But it can do what you just described, namely help you not be consumed by your pain and find a lighter approach of handling it.
Maya:	*(nods)*
Therapist:	You see, whatever we pay attention to tends to become bigger in our heads. This is true for a simple meditation exercise like this one, and it's true for your pain. But it also matters the way in which we pay attention: we can focus rigidly on something and judge it harshly, or we can focus flexibly and just observe without judgment. It's hard, but it's possible. And it's a skill everyone can learn.
Maya:	But I will never not hate my pain. It just makes my life so miserable.
Therapist:	I understand. Unfortunately, nothing I can do will make this pain disappear. But you have just experienced what it means to carry your pain with more lightness. And if you practice your focus in a different way like we did just now, you can learn to carry it with more lightness, and you can have your life back.

Maya: I just don't want to be in pain.

Therapist: I hear you. And if I could wave a wand to make it disappear, I would. Unfortunately, your body has changed. And now it's up to you to get to know this new body of yours: what you are truly capable of, and how you can get your life back. Does this sound like a worthwhile goal?

Maya: Yes. I want to do that.

Therapist: Great! What we just practiced takes a while to get used to, but it offers health benefits if you practice it regularly. It's not about erasing pain, but about getting more in tune with your body, and creating more lightness in dealing with difficult feelings. Would you be willing to give this practice a try at home?

In this conversation segment, the therapist taught Maya a fundamental mindfulness practice. By practicing awareness in this way, Maya can learn to focus her attention in a more flexible and less judgmental way that allows for more variation and more flexible selection. With repeated practice, Maya will be able to direct her attention more deliberately, rather than being pushed around by her pain. Note that the aim here is not to change the experience itself: it's not about diminishing her pain, but about lessening the influence the pain has on Maya, her actions, and her overall level of experienced anger.

The therapist has invited Maya to mindfully observe her experience whenever her mind wanders into difficult territory. In other words, whenever Maya notices that she gets fearful of reinjuring herself, or when she notices her mind being caught up in worry or anger, or when she focuses rigidly on her pain, she is meant to use these moments as opportunities to practice mindfulness. If we add the new element "Mindfulness practice" (together with its underlying relations to other factors) to Maya's network model, it might look similar to what we can see in figure 7.2. Notice that the arrowheads originating from "Mindfulness practice" are hollow, so as to indicate that these relations diminish the strength of their attached factors.

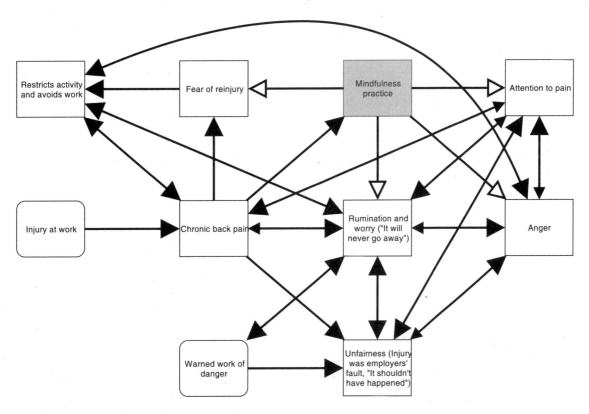

Figure 7.2 Effect of Maya's mindfulness practice

The mindfulness practice allows Maya to relate to her body in a more aware, compassionate way. Instead of being dominated by painful thoughts, feelings, and sensations, Maya can choose her focus and connect with what is really there (rather than mindlessly believe what her mind tells her). In this way, the therapist and Maya addressed one key factor that adds to Maya's anger. However, there remain other key factors responsible for Maya's anger, which need to be addressed as well. And it's these other factors that we turn to next.

Maya's thoughts tend to circle around her pain—that it "may never go away," that her injury was "unfair," and that it "shouldn't have happened." These thoughts, while possibly true, add to her anger because they paint Maya as the victim of a meaningless tragedy. In her view, life has played a mean trick on her, and there's nothing she can do about it. As long as Maya continues to cling to these unhelpful thoughts, real change is unlikely to happen. For this reason, the therapist needs to address Maya's sense of self-efficacy and put her back in the driver's seat, where she can start believing in her ability to steer the course of her life.

As you can see in Maya's network model (figure 7.2), there are several factors that reinforce Maya's tendency to worry and ruminate. Unfortunately, no therapist in the world will be able to undo the injury that resulted in her back pain. Nor will they be able to change the fact that Maya's superiors neglected her warnings, thus leading Maya to believe her accident was "unfair." It is now up to Maya to find a different way of responding to these unchangeable realities—a way that allows for more flexibility so that next to her self-defeating thoughts is also space for self-empowering ones. Building a client's sense of self-efficacy is a long-term process, where the client has to create incremental experiences of setting and achieving self-chosen goals. In this way, the client's belief in their own capability can grow.

Nonetheless, it's possible to spark this process by showing the client that they can go beyond the limitations they set on themselves. Below is an example of what this can look like.

Therapist: I would like to do a different exercise. For this exercise you can leave your eyes open, you can stay in your seat, and we only need one arm. Sounds good?

Maya: Ahem, yes, I guess.

Therapist: Alright, for this exercise, I would like you to pick an arm, and then raise it up as high as possible without leaving your seat. You got it?

Maya: Yes, I cannot lift it anymore.

Therapist: You are as high as you can get?

Maya: Yes.

Therapist: Great. And now, see if you can lift it just a millimeter more. Excellent. Very good. You can now put your arm back down. The point of this silly exercise is to show that what our mind says must not necessarily be true. You said you cannot lift your arm any more. But when I asked you to lift your arm even higher, you were able to do it.

Maya: I don't understand. What does this have to do with me?

Therapist: It seems that your mind has come up with some very strict thoughts that what happened to you is unfair, and that it will never get away, and that you can't do anything anymore. Is this right?

Maya: Well, yes, but that's all true.

Therapist: It can be. Yes. And then again, it might not be. What if, just like lifting your arm, you can do more than your mind tells you that you can? You might not be able to do everything in the same way as before the accident. And yes, your pain might never fully go away. But what if you have untapped potential? What if you have possibilities that your mind does not yet see because it's too focused on the fact that your pain may never go away?

Maya: I'm limiting myself too much.

Therapist: Maybe. It's up to us to discover what this untapped potential can be. I'd like to explore this with you more in-depth together. It will require getting in touch with yourself more, and rather than just believing the limitations your mind tells you, really feeling into your body and exploring your true new range.

In the above conversation segment, the therapist added an element of self-efficacy to Maya's network model. As previously mentioned, for self-efficacy to grow a steadfast hold in Maya's life, she will have to do more than just one quick exercise with her therapist. Building self-efficacy is a long-term process of setting and achieving self-chosen goals (or living by self-chosen commitments and values). The more consistent the client can be in this endeavor, the more solid their sense of self-efficacy can become. Despite the small nature of the exercise, it demonstrated to Maya that the limits of her mind do not necessarily reflect her true limitations, and that she has the potential to go beyond what she formerly believed was possible. By empowering Maya to start believing in her ability to affect meaningful change in her life, two crucial things can happen: First, Maya stops being the victim of her circumstances and becomes an active agent in her life once again, thus decreasing her sense of felt anger (which partially stemmed from her presumed felt powerlessness). Second, since an increased sense of self-efficacy diminishes the influence of her chronic back pain on her life, Maya is less likely to ruminate and worry about her pain. Maya may notice that although life might not go back to the way it was, she is still capable of living her life with intention and purpose. By introducing this powerful new element in Maya's life, other changes might get easier to come by. If we add this new element of self-efficacy (as well as its underlying relations) to Maya's network model, it might look similar to what we can see in figure 7.3.

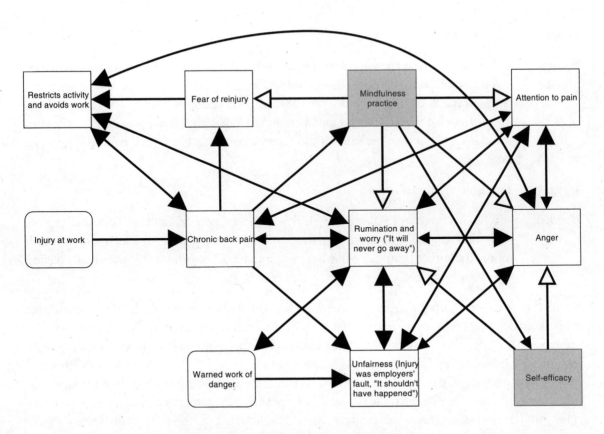

Figure 7.3 Effect of Maya's self-efficacy

By now, Maya has established two new adaptive elements in her network model (i.e., "Mindfulness practice" and "Self-efficacy"), both of which pull from her maladaptive processes and allow for greater variation and more flexible selection (meaning Maya has more options available of how she can choose to react in her situation). The therapist has put Maya back in a position where she can get more in tune with her own body and start believing in her ability to affect meaningful change in her life. As a result, it's now time to figure out what this meaning can be. In the following conversation we will play this out.

Maya: Sometimes it gets easier to go through my day, but the pain is always there. And sometimes it's just all I can think about.

Therapist: This may sound like an odd question, but what if the pain was gone?

Maya: What do you mean? That would be wonderful, of course.

Therapist: I'm sure it would. But what I specifically mean is what would you do if you didn't have pain?

Maya: I don't know. I haven't really thought about it. I mean it doesn't matter either way, because the pain is there—whether I want it or not.

Therapist: I understand. And from what I can tell you pretty much put your entire life on hold when the pain came into your life. Is that true?

Maya: (*Tearing up*) It's made me so miserable.

Therapist: I hear you. Your pain has made many things much more difficult for you, or even straight out impossible. And still: You are still breathing. There's still a life in here that wants to be lived. And I'm willing to bet that there are still things in life that you care about—regardless of whether or not you are in pain.

Maya: That's true. Very true.

Therapist: Alright. So suppose a miracle happens and your pain disappears. I'm not saying it will, but for the sake of this exercise, let's just pretend it will. And in a few years from now, you would be interviewed on live television about how you handled yourself and what you were like when you were going through the worst. In the ideal world, what would you like yourself to say?

Maya: I guess I'd like myself to say that I was...um...loving...and kind toward myself. And... um...patient and hopeful.

Therapist: Anything else?

Maya: That I didn't give up. And that I was there for other people as well.

Therapist: So to be loving, kind, patient, and hopeful. And that you continue to be there for yourself and for others.

Maya: Yeah.

Therapist: Okay, so just sit with this for a moment. To be loving, kind, patient, hopeful, and supportive: that's what matters to you.

Maya: Yes. I want to do what's best for myself, but I also want to help others. I have several friends at work, and they have to deal with the same mess that got me here in the first place.

Therapist: Okay. So next time you notice yourself ruminating and worrying about your pain, "whether it will go away," or that "all of it was unfair," it seems that you have a choice. You can let your mind bully you, and let your pain push you around and tell you what to do or not to do. Or, alternatively, you can choose to not engage these unhelpful thoughts, and instead focus on what is truly important here, namely being loving, kind, patient, hopeful, and supportive. You can be the sort of person you want to be, despite pain and difficult thoughts showing up. Which of these two options will you choose?

Maya: Well, I want to be loving and hopeful and supportive.

Therapist: Great. If it's okay for you, I would like to use our remaining time to explore what living by these values—loving, hopeful, and supportive—would look like, and how you can bring these values into your life.

In the conversation, the therapist explored with Maya what would make her life worth living. Maya has built her entire life around her pain, and now it's time for her to build a life that includes her pain but doesn't make it the central focus. It became clear that Maya values being loving, kind, patient, hopeful, and supportive of both herself and others. Subsequently, it is up to Maya and the therapist to explore how she can bring these values into her life and translate them into real actions and achievable goals or commitments. Although a new focus on what matters to Maya doesn't necessarily strip away her rumination and worries, it does strengthen her sense of self-efficacy, since she is now more in touch with her core motivations. Furthermore, this new focus on what she values might diminish her fear of reinjury, since her chronic back pain stands less and less in the center of her life, thus making the risk of reinjury seem less scary. If we add the new element "Focus on valued goals" (together with its underlying relations to other factors) to Maya's network model, it might look similar to what we can see in figure 7.4. Notice that "Mindfulness practice" strengthens Maya's focus on valued goals, since mindful awareness fosters an overall self-awareness, including of what she values.

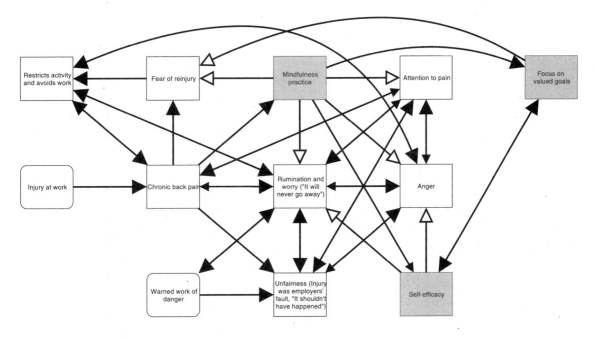

Figure 7.4 Effect of Maya's focus on valued goals

As the therapy progresses, more and more elements get introduced to Maya's network model that reduce maladaptive processes. As you can see, those new elements are set up in a self-reinforcing way: the node "Mindfulness practice" reinforces the nodes "Focus on valued goals" and "Self-efficacy"— both of which also reinforce each other. In this way, step by step, adaptive loops get introduced and become more dominant. In the following section, we will expand Maya's focus on what matters to her by turning her values into actionable commitments. In other words, we will work on retention by solidifying new responses into full habits.

HOW TO INCREASE RETENTION

Retention is about making positive changes stick. Oftentimes, maladaptive responses have been solidified through self-reinforcing loops. Maladaptation fosters maladaptation. The longer the client has been stuck in such a pattern, the more their responses have turned into rigid habits, and the harder it is for the client to make a change.

Retention is the opposite: repeating a positive pattern and building it into larger integrated patterns. That can happen with any of the dimensions of the EEMM: repeating adaptive attentional strategies helps retain them; building healthy cognitive processes into large patterns of adjustment does likewise; and so on. The strongest and most certain route to retention, however, is linking positive processes of change to positively motivated overt behavior. Creating a life worth living is where the rubber meets the road.

Retention thus involves linking processes of change to adaptive responses and experimenting with different strategies to turn them into sustainable habits that cluster into larger patterns of action. Given that goal, a key to retention is adopting a new response that makes sense within the client's network model. It is ideal if the new pattern acts as an alternative to a maladaptive one. For instance, Maya's tendency to restrict herself from activities and work is fostering her anger and exacerbating her pain and rumination. By connecting a new response to other established nodes—such as her focus on valued goals—it becomes more sustainable.

Some clients will require little assistance in selecting strategies for retaining a new response, while others may need all the help you can lend. There is no rule of thumb that works for everyone, and instead it will come down to a process of experimentation. Discuss a course of action, give the client time to implement it, reconvene and reflect, and ultimately adapt the course of action to better serve the client's interest. Here is an example of how the process of choosing and retaining a new response played out with Maya.

Therapist: We have talked about you wanting to be loving, patient, and supportive. Let's talk a bit about what this means, and how you can bring these values into your life. For instance, what does it mean for you to be "loving"?

Maya: I guess treating myself better. Being more kind to myself. Being nicer to my soul and body.

Therapist: And how could you do that?

Maya: By giving myself what I need. For example, I know I have been putting off some exercises my physical therapist and physician have recommended to me. I know I need to do it. I just don't.

Therapist: So one way to be more loving to yourself would be to start exercising?!

Maya: Yes, I think so.

Therapist: Can you tell me about the exercises?

Maya: The biggest thing would be stretching exercises. Something like yoga. I even bought myself a mat, but I never used it.

Therapist: Okay, so you know the type of exercises you should be doing, and you have the equipment you need.

Maya: Yeah.

Therapist: What stands in the way?

Maya: It's bit scary, to be honest. I'm scared of hurting myself. My doc says no, but I still fear it. And then there's follow through. Will I even do it?

Therapist: Fear will need to be part of it at first. It sounds to me that you've been listening to your fear. This is pretty much what you have been doing for a while, and while it's understandable, you know from experience how this affects you. Your life becomes smaller, and your pain actually becomes bigger, no? What if we listened instead to being there for yourself in a loving, patient, and supportive way. And one way to do that is by exercising. You can get your life back and give your body what it needs. If you have these two choices sitting on the table in front of your, which would you choose?

Maya: The second one. Exercising.

Therapist: Great. Now on a level of 1 to 10, how certain are you that you will actually do the exercises your physical trainer had recommended?

Maya: I'm not sure. Maybe a 6?

Therapist: Alright, a 6 is not too bad. Now I would like to raise your level of certainty, at least to an 8 or a 9. One thing that helps many people is having someone else, so you can do exercises together. Do you have someone you could ask?

Maya: I have a neighbor who I'm friendly with, and he is doing yoga every morning. I could ask him to exercise together.

Therapist: Great. And if you do that, how would you rate your level of certainty? It's alright if it didn't change, but if it did, where would you put it?

Maya: Well, then it's definitely a 9.

Therapist: Great. So your plan is to ask your neighbor about exercising together in the morning, and then we talk again next time about how it went. Willing?

Maya: I'm willing.

The therapist and Maya did two things: First, they explored alternative responses to maladaptive responses. And second, they explored strategies to increase Maya's odds of following through with the new responses. Maya has chosen to act on her value of being self-loving by doing the stretching exercises her physical trainer had recommended to her. And in order to increase her odds of following through, Maya has committed herself to ask her neighbor for additional social support.

Maya's new course of action is motivated by her values, and it is reinforced by other established parts in Maya's network. Later on in Maya's case, the therapist again used the "broaden and build" strategy of creating adaptive habits to compete with difficult emotions. Since pain, a sense of unfairness, and anger could still disrupt the new pattern, the therapist took advantage of a new opportunity to apply the progress Maya has made to a new area.

Maya: The situation at work is still a mess, and I kind of worry about my friends and coworkers there. The folks in charge have no idea about the conditions at work, and someone needs to fix it. It's just wrong.

Therapist: Can I ask? If you take that same core value—being loving and supportive—is there any place you can put that motivation when you see that unfairness at work? Is there a way to support to your friends and coworkers?

Maya: I always wanted to join the worker's union. You know, make a difference so that what happened to me doesn't happen to anyone else.

Therapist: And how would you do that?

Maya: I'm not sure exactly how it works, but I know someone who is in the union, so I could ask her. I've had it in the back of my mind for a long time.

Therapist: Cool. And you would be willing to do that before our next session?

Maya: Definitely. It's easier than exercising and I did that!

The extent to which it is necessary to explore strategies to increase the client's odds of successfully retaining gains will vary based on the client, their unique context, and the intended change. Here Maya's progress came in part from deciding to act on her values and becoming active in a worker's union, which applies that same motivation and gives her a positive place to put her feeling of unfairness. Both sets of responses—participating in the worker's union and exercising with her neighbor—are supporting Maya's belief in her ability to affect change. Both diminish the risk for relapse posed by Maya's overall sense of felt anger and a sense of unfairness. Maya's anger fueled her decision to participate in the worker's union, but by becoming active in this way, her anger (or the dominance of her anger) lessened (hence the double-headed excitatory-inhibitory relation).

If we add these new elements of "Participate in worker's union" and "Morning exercise with neighbor" (together with their underlying relations to other factors), it might look similar to what we can see in figure 7.5.

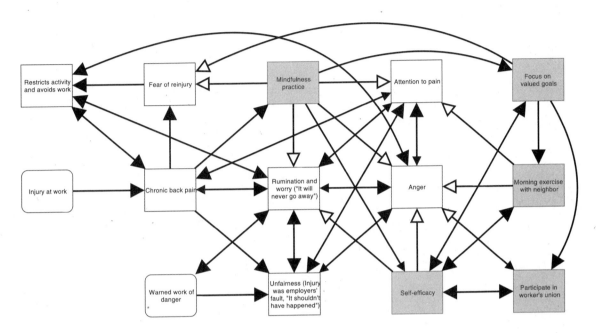

Figure 7.5 Effect of Maya's morning exercise
with neighbor and participation in worker's union

By introducing new strategies to deal with her problems, Maya's network model might be able to now shift in a fundamental way. Rather than being stuck in self-reinforcing loops of maladaptation, central factors are now in place that could reinforce adaptive responses and adaptive loops instead. As a result, her overall anger could diminish.

Maya has not been able to get rid of her chronic pain, nor was she able to completely shut off negative thoughts and feelings around her pain and injury. But if she's successful, Maya will utilize new, more adaptive ways of responding to her reality. Rather than being the victim of her circumstances, Maya will become empowered to actively shape her life in meaningful ways.

However, as we will see in chapter 11, these are mere predictions that need to be evaluated. If these predictions are incorrect and the strategies do not have the intended effects on the network, even after repeated attempts, the therapist needs to be prepared to flexibly adjust the approach. We will revisit Maya again in chapter 11 when we discuss the course of treatment. There we will illustrate how to incorporate data in the treatment process to examine the validity of the hypothesized network and then how to reorient and reconsider the approach and apply suitable therapeutic techniques in a flexible manner in a given context.

Action Step 7.1 Fill in the Your Complete EEMM

Let's return to the problem you identified in your own life. Based on previous action steps (especially Action Steps 4.3, 4.4, 6.3, and 6.4), see if you can fill in a full EEMM below as it relates to your problem, focusing primarily on maladaptive processes. Remember that retention and contextual control may touch on issues in other rows (i.e., dimensions and levels).

	Variation	Selection	Retention	Context
Affect				
Cognition				
Attention				
Self				

	Variation	Selection	Retention	Context
Motivation				
Overt Behavior				
Biophysiological				
Sociocultural				

Example

	Variation	Selection	Retention	Context
Affect	I turn down social situations that might make me anxious.	I immediately feel better, but I also soon fear the next situation.	My fear grows stronger whenever I buy into it and escape it.	It gets reinforced by my history, my focus, and my actions.
Cognition	I think that I will embarrass myself, and people will not like me.	I get a sense of control if I am just vigilant enough.	Regardless of how others react, I have to stay vigilant of not embarrassing myself.	It gets reinforced by my history and my actions.
Attention	I watch out for signs of impending anxiety.	I feel safer and less vulnerable, even if it interferes with my performance.	Regardless of what happens, I need to stay vigilant to make sure I don't embarrass myself.	It gets reinforced by my history, my emotions, and body sensations.
Self	I think of myself as a "loser" and "not good enough."	By rejecting myself first, I soften the rejection by others.	I only make experiences that confirm my self-perception.	It gets reinforced by my history, my actions, and my focus.
Motivation	I'm primarily concerned with not embarrassing myself. I want others to like me.	I want to feel safe and appreciated.	Regardless of how others react, I have to stay vigilant of not embarrassing myself.	It gets reinforced by my history, my actions, and my focus.

	Variation	Selection	Retention	Context
Overt Behavior	I overcompensate and try to be funny, or I retreat home.	I want to be liked, or I want to avoid feeling hurt from rejection.	Regardless of how others react, I have to prove myself or escape my pain.	It gets reinforced by my feelings, my self-perception, and my motivation.
Biophysiological	My stomach tightens, my heart beats faster, I begin to get fidgety.	My body prepares for imminent danger.	These sensations grow stronger when I escape my fear.	It gets reinforced by my feelings, my actions, and my thoughts.
Sociocultural	I learned in high school that there are "winners and losers."	Clinging to these black/white terms gives me a false sense of security.	These beliefs get reinforced whenever I act on them.	It gets reinforced by my actions, my history, and my feelings.

Thus far in the book, we've covered the tools central to process-based therapy: the network approach and the EEMM, including its six psychological dimensions (cognition, affect, attention, self, motivation, and overt behavior), two levels (biophysiological and sociocultural), and four critical characteristics (variation, selection, context, and retention). We've applied these tools to clinical cases and, through action steps, to a problem you identified in your own life. At this point, we are going to take a closer look at the processes of change, the mechanisms necessary for treatment to be successful.

CHAPTER 8

A Closer Look at Processes

The processes in a client's life shape and determine their reality. When the processes are adaptive, the client moves closer to their goals and aspirations, on a path to a healthy, happy, and fulfilling life. When the processes are maladaptive, however, the client moves off course, engages in self-destructive habits, and invites pain, misery, and regret into their life. In process-based therapy, we aim to help the client disrupt old maladaptive processes and instead build new adaptive processes that serve their deeper and more meaningful interests.

We have already talked about the role of processes in the development of clinical struggles, but now it's time to look at processes in the context of therapy. Which process should be targeted with which therapeutic intervention? How can you measure relevant processes and track their progression? How does a functional analysis change when the processes within it change? And how can you build new adaptive processes into self-sustaining networks?

We will address these questions and more over the following pages. And we will do so by returning to the case of Julie. As you might remember, Julie has a hard time standing up for herself. Her mother tried molding her into a "nice girl," and now she often resorts to people pleasing. She genuinely wants to help people, which inspired her career, but she also often stands in her own way of enforcing her needs and boundaries without feeling selfish.

Julie has a husband who is frequently unsupportive, which further reinforces her tendency to avoid difficult conversations altogether. In figure 8.1, you can see Julie's network model. At the center of Julie's clinical situation is her struggle to stand up for herself, which is reinforced by an array of other factors, and further feeds into her maladaptive beliefs, behaviors, and relationship dynamics. The goal in therapy is then to introduce new adaptive factors and disrupt old maladaptive ones, so that Julie can better enforce her own needs and boundaries. We'll explore ways to do this using the EEMM grid, which we'll introduce next.

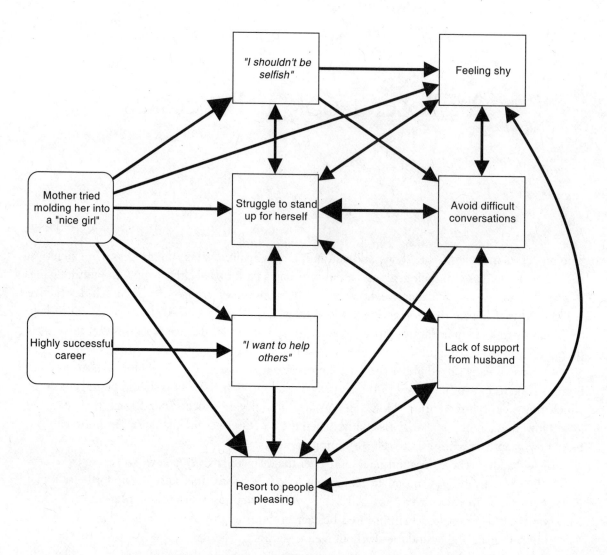

Figure 8.1 Revisiting Julie's network model

THE EEMM GRID

The benefits of the Extended Evolutionary Meta-Model (EEMM) for process-based therapy (PBT) are especially obvious in the stage of process-based functional analysis. The EEMM reminds us as practitioners to consider how to instigate change, how to recognize positive steps as they occur, how to promote maintenance of these steps in the right direction, and to make sure that skills that are learned fit the challenges of the internal and external situation. The EEMM also nudges us as practitioners to keep our eyes wide, considering relevant psychological dimensions and biophysiological and sociocultural levels of analysis.

That first set of questions—the columns of the EEMM—are answered by the dynamic relationship among elements in the case. Said in another way, if we've picked the key nodes and relations, that first set of questions is answered by the network itself. But notice the word "if"—how can we be reminded to do a better job of picking the key nodes and relations?

In the rest of the book, we will use a device that we think helps. It has the great benefit of creating more consistency in how we use networks to do process-based functional analysis, while also providing a reminder and a positive nudge for selecting features of the case to track. Take a look at figure 8.2.

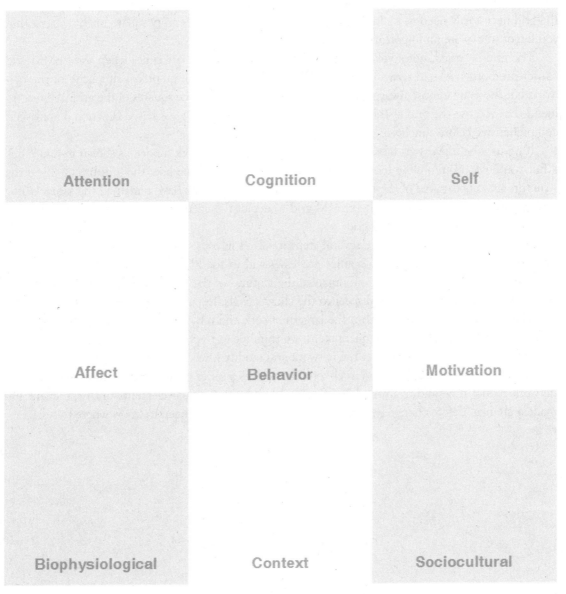

Figure 8.2 The EEMM grid

The EEMM grid is a shaded template comprising squares that represent the various dimensions and levels of EEMM. The purpose of the grid is to derive a consistent network for a particular client. This grid will enable different clinicians (regardless of their therapeutic orientation) to derive the same (or a very similar) network of a client's problem. For this, it is important to use the client's own words describing the problem (rather than interpreting the client's report early on) and to be as concrete as possible (i.e., ask about actual events, thoughts, behaviors, and so on). This information represents the key nodes of the problem, including any moderators and other contextual factors, the six psychological dimensions, and the biophysiological and sociocultural levels. This grid will help you keep the EEMM in the back of your mind as you develop the client's network. Not all squares of the grid necessarily need to include a node for every client, but an empty square might suggest that you forgot to explore an important dimension.

The grid is an aid, not a yoke to put around your neck. There are times when the EEMM grid can create bottlenecks in terms of placement of the nodes and the graphical simplicity of the network, but those are almost always solvable simply by repositioning the squares of the grid. We recommend that you use the grid at the initial stage to make sure the process-based functional analysis is comprehensive before simplifying it.

If we use the EEMM grid for Julie's case, it will shift her network model, as shown in figure 8.3. After you have taken a close look, compare it to figure 8.1, and see how the grid has changed the structure and appearance of the model while the nodes and arrows have remained the same. Going forward, we will continue using the EEMM grid to depict the client's network models, placing each node in the applicable area of the grid.

As you might recall, there are several steps involved in a process-based diagnosis. These steps involve having a model that can organize processes within the EEMM and then homing in on the processes themselves. This means we organize the features of the network into known change processes and moderators—all with respect to the client's goals. In particular, we focus on self-amplifying relations and subnetworks within the larger network and rely, wherever possible, on empirically established relationships. In subsequent steps, we then measure processes and outcomes as needed, and, based on that data, reconsider the network and modify it where necessary. Process-based functional analysis, which we described in chapter 3, involves a series of steps that require revisiting the network model time and again and twisting and turning individual elements until the client has made a change. Before change becomes possible, however, we first need to know where to start.

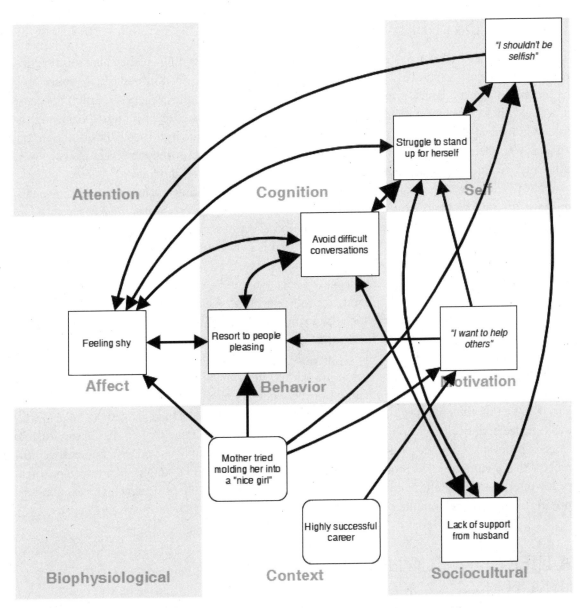

Figure 8.3 Julie's network model with the EEMM grid

IDENTIFYING RELEVANT PROCESSES

The processes in a network model are not equally important. Depending on the client's difficulties, needs, and wishes, some processes play a more central role, while others not so much. A process may be central because it is largely responsible for maintaining and facilitating a client's struggle or because it actively hinders the client from progressing toward their goals and deeper interests. Knowing the role of individual processes will not only give you important insights into the client's situation, but also tell you where you can best start with therapeutic interventions. Although processes will always differ between individual clients, there are helpful rules of thumb you can follow.

The processes in a network model come in two varieties: originating and maintaining. *Originating processes* are important in explaining how a problem came to be, while *maintaining processes* are important in explaining what upholds it. In working with a client, we are interested in both. Nonetheless, as important as it may be to understand how a struggle arose, it is more vital to know what maintains it. By uncovering maintaining processes, we get a better understanding of the client's current situation and gain the knowledge we need to disrupt and diminish their difficulties. Originating processes, on the other hand, are only relevant to the degree that they speak to the current situation. Therefore, we put the focus on maintaining processes.

In Julie's case, for instance, her mother had tried molding her into a "nice girl," which put her on a path toward people pleasing. While it certainly explains how Julie came to have this particular problem, it cannot be undone since there is no way to interfere with the past. This is the unfortunate reality of any client dealing with difficult past experiences. Nonetheless, we can interfere in the present, by targeting the processes that maintain Julie's struggles. For instance, by getting Julie to willingly engage in difficult conversations and practice her ability to stand up for herself, she can learn to let go of people pleasing—regardless of any past experience she might have had with her mother. Any process that maintains Julie's problems in the present moment might be suitable as a target for therapeutic interventions as long as it leads to adaptation. In short, when choosing which process to prioritize in therapy, pick maintaining processes.

A HIERARCHY OF PROCESSES AND THE "UNCHANGEABLE CLIENT"

Some processes encompass others. For example, self-compassion can be thought of as a single process, but it can also be deconstructed into self-kindness, mindfulness, and a sense of common humanity—the acknowledgment that suffering is part of the human experience. In the same way, these deconstructed processes can then be further deconstructed into even smaller parts. This ladder of ever smaller subprocesses is called the *hierarchy of processes*. When you look at a client's network model, look out for *process supersets*—umbrellas under which minor processes are functioning—and then deconstruct them into smaller processes.

By deconstructing a superset, you can do more justice to the client's experience by painting their case with the necessary complexity and depth. More importantly, doing so will give you a therapeutic advantage when larger ways of being get in the way of what the client needs from you. Some processes may have become so ingrained in a client's way of being that they seem beyond any clinical intervention. Once these processes have been deconstructed, however, you may begin to see an opening point in a subprocess that is susceptible to change. In this manner, bit by bit, you can work your way up to the larger process.

For instance, suppose a client adheres to a political and cultural ideology that emphasizes being in control but has relationship problems that come from that very pattern. It may be ineffective to challenge the entire belief system, but by deconstructing the larger pattern you may see that it consists of individual practices, only some of which are interfering with the client's goals. Some of that subset, in turn, may be fairly susceptible to change.

The classic movie *American History X* provides a kind of example. Actor Edward Norton portrayed a neo-Nazi who strictly adhered to an ideology of hate and violence. However, after befriending an African American inmate and becoming a target for the Aryan Brotherhood, he slowly began to distance himself from his hateful beliefs. It wasn't an overnight change, but a gradual one, and his core beliefs where challenged—bit by bit—through new experiences, each experience chipping away at the pillars that upheld his ideology. Although changes like these are rare, they happen, and they always start in small, inconspicuous ways.

In a similar way, hierarchies of maladaptive processes may gather into patterns that are spoken of as if the client cannot change ("personality disorders" would be the classic and common example). A process-focused approach provides a useful route forward in such cases.

ACCESSIBILITY OF PROCESSES OF CHANGE

As an extension of this same thinking, some processes are better suited to be targeted in therapy simply because they are more directly accessible, the client is more willing to work in this area, and changes in processes in one area set up healthy changes in another. For instance, a client may have a deep-seated belief that she is worthless due to an abuse history. A frontal intervention on this core belief may be impractical because the client will waive it off, and it may be unhelpful because the client dissociates when the history is addressed directly. Instead, working on, say, distress tolerance skills may be more accessible and may set up the more difficult work down the road. This is the reason why we identify the hierarchy of processes in the first place: because deconstructing process supersets into subprocesses makes them more accessible.

There are certain criteria that determine whether a process is accessible. Can you reach a process with therapeutic interventions? Do you have permission from the client? Do you have the required technical knowledge? Is the setting and the kind of work allowing you to do it? All these questions need to be considered when you inquire about the accessibility. You may deal with a client whose cultural process is bound up by a belief system that they do not like looking at. You might have permission to work with a client on their emotions, but not on their childhood history. Sometimes the barrier is the client's limit and it needs to be addressed directly (e.g., "We are going to have to deal with XYZ or we will not be able to make progress"). In other cases, the barrier is in the situation, such as when insurance doesn't cover a certain treatment program or focus. Whatever the barrier may be, it is important to identify it and find ways to work around it.

MEASURING RELEVANT PROCESSES

In therapy, you need to know where you are going. You need to know whether you are actually helping the client make progress toward their goals or whether you are just spinning your wheels. Only with reliable feedback will you be able to tell which of these two is accurate, which is why you need to track important processes.

As we already discussed, you want to focus on processes that are central to the client's issues and accessible with clinical interventions. After you have found a process that fulfills these criteria, you have to home in on a particular aspect of this process. For instance, a client who frequently overeats in order to cope with thoughts of worthlessness might be best helped by monitoring their self-defeating thoughts. Although this work might be more complex than just the tracking of self-defeating thoughts, if their functional impact is central to the client's maladaptive behavior (i.e., overeating), they need to be tracked. The same might not be true with a different client dealing with the same problem. Network analysis and idiographic assessment will help you pick relevant processes that make most sense to track.

The measurement method should be reliable and convenient for the client, thus increasing the odds that the resulting data will be both accurate and useful. A popular measurement method is self-report, but we need to get beyond extensive, psychometrically based instruments that can only be utilized periodically and move toward single-item or very short measures that can be taken frequently and linked to content. Some of these can be generated by taking items with high factor loading in existing tests. A wide variety of such measures are becoming available. Assessment intervals have to be short enough to estimate within-person variability but infrequent enough and covering a long enough time span that they capture meaningful sequences without becoming a burden for the client.

In-session behaviors are a ready source of information. Advances in automatic generation and scoring of therapy transcripts is making assessment of client word choice in therapy a readily available option, and already we know they may be used to assess important processes of change (Hesser at al., 2009). Simple biophysiological measures, often with smartphone connections, are also available.

Let's return now to Julie. Central to her difficulties are her struggle to stand up for herself, her tendency to avoid difficult conversations, and her habit of people pleasing at the cost of self-care. These factors all currently contribute to keeping her stuck, and they all spin around the axis of her thoughts of being selfish. In the following conversation segment, the therapist will recommend tracking her self-defeating thoughts and will suggest a method of how this can best be done.

NOTICING JULIE'S THOUGHTS

Therapist: It seems that your thoughts and the way you think about yourself play an important role in your struggle to stand up for yourself. Would that be fair to say?

Julie: Yes, that's probably right. I just can't help it.

Therapist: I know, thoughts can be very tricky. It's sometimes as if our thoughts have a mind of their own. They just come and go as they please, without much regard for whether we actually want them or not.

Julie: Yes, it sometimes does feel that way.

Therapist: So I'm not trying to tell you to stop thinking whatever you are thinking, because that's not how our minds work. Instead, I'd like to know exactly how often your mind turns to these thoughts that make it hard for you to standup for yourself. Are you with me?

Julie: Yes. So what are we going to do?

Therapist: I have a mission for you for the next week. I would like to take a peek inside your world to see how your mind raises issues of "selfishness" and whether that thought and ones like it make it hard for you to stand up for yourself. These can be any thoughts where you talk badly about yourself or where you discourage yourself from maintaining a healthy boundary.

Julie: Okay, I think I could do that.

Therapist: Great! Now I want it to be as easy as possible for you, so you don't have to run around everywhere with a pen and notebook in your hand. Do you have your phone with you most of the time?

Julie: Yes, I never go anywhere without it. *(laughs)*

Therapist: Great. There is a simple app I use that will ping you about four to five times a day between whatever times we set. I'll send you the link and we can change it, but right now it's set for 9 a.m. to 9 p.m. When it pings, I just want you to say if you've had the thought *I'm selfish* over the last ten minutes and, if so, how believable that thought was using a scale from "not at all" to "completely." If you had any other thought that makes it hard for you to stand up for yourself, you can enter that one too and rate it for believ-ability. Finally, it will ask if right now you are alone or with someone and whether you are having a conversation about anything of importance to you, positive or negative. Does this sound doable to you? It's should take less than sixty seconds to do, four or five times a day.

Julie: Yes, I think I can do that. I will probably skip a few if it catches me at a really bad time, but I'll give it a try.

Therapist: Great! And that's no problem is you have to skip a couple. Just see if you can do most of them. Just these kinds of thoughts and how they land for next seven days.

If you use this type of tool, make sure to give the client a good justification for using it so they understand why and what you are going to measure.

One good thing about self-monitoring like this is that measurement itself can motivate change. Julie may find it easier to stand up for herself and engage in difficult conversations merely by becom-ing more conscious of her thought process and knowing that her therapist will track these relation-ships. Instead of mindlessly following the commands of her historically produced thoughts, Julie can create some healthy distance between herself and her thinking, loosening the grip of self-critical thoughts like *I shouldn't be selfish.* All of these factors (e.g., "Avoid difficult conversations," "Struggle to stand up for herself") trigger self-defeating thoughts and thus give Julie a reason to record them (hence the relationship in this direction is excitatory).

If we add "Record self-defeating thoughts" as a new node (along with its relations to other nodes) in Julie's network model, placing it in the cognition dimension of the grid, it will look similar to what you can see in figure 8.4.

This new node in Julie's network model will not only give us better insights into her problems (since we get a better picture of the type of thoughts that trouble Julie, as well as of their frequency), but also introduce an adaptive twist in Julie's established processes. In this way, a method of measure-ment can simultaneously be an intervention. This is not true of all methods of measurement. In the next therapy session, it is up to Julie and the therapist to take the newly acquired knowledge and adjust their approach accordingly. This is where mediators come in.

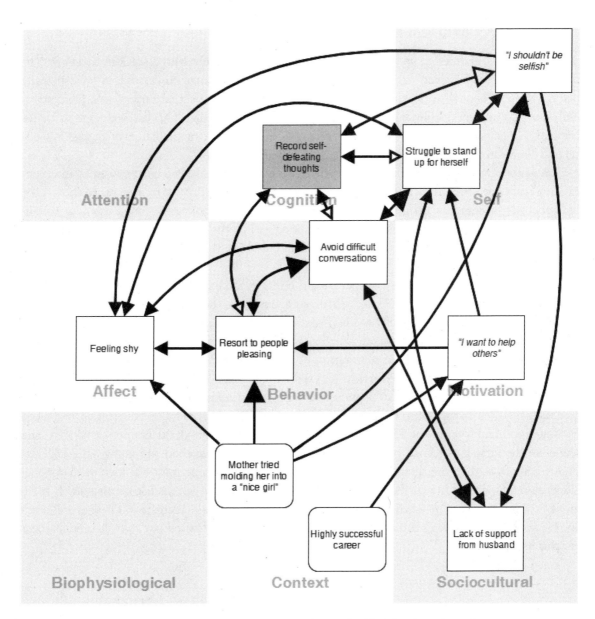

Figure 8.4 Effect of Julie's recording of self-defeating thoughts

SELECTING MEDIATORS

There are countless different approaches you can take to help a client who is stuck in their ways. To make things easier, however, we have compiled a partial list of change processes that are especially helpful when a client is stuck in a specific dimension (cognition, affect, attention, self, motivation, and behavior) or level (biophysiological or sociocultural) of the EEMM. This list of change processes is based on a massive meta-analysis of the world's scientific literature on mediators of change in mental and behavioral health (Hayes, Hofmann, Ciarrochi, et al., 2020).

Mediators are functionally important pathways to outcomes that have been moved by intervention and that have been shown to relate to outcomes when controlling for treatment. In short, they are processes of change with proven treatment utility. We have jokingly named this large meta-analysis of mediators the Deathstar Project, because, just like the artificial planet in the Star Wars movies, the project was gigantic, took forever to build, and, we think, can severely disrupt ongoing activities.

We included all bona fide psychotherapeutic intervention/experimental studies, as well as all psychotherapeutic orientations and major therapeutic outcomes that identified significant mediators in randomized trials of psychosocial methods as compared to treatment as usual or no treatment. Using very broad search criteria, we identified nearly 55,000 potential mediational studies. Multiple raters conducted abstract screenings, resulting in nearly 110,000 independent ratings from which they identified approximately 1,500 articles that potentially meet criteria for mediation.

After we spent a long time reading and categorizing the studies, the following table came to light (see table 8.1). You can see which change process was most frequently found to be effective, organized by dimension and level of the EEMM. Note that the Deathstar Project is not yet concluded, and therefore the table is not final. Nor is the table exhaustive, because there are many more effective change processes than are shown here. We merely depicted the three most effective mediators per dimension and level as are currently indicated by our data (leaving out mediators that simply mentioned the label of the row—such as studies showing that "affect" was a mediator). These are all listed in the words of each study's authors, by the way, so we have not imposed our own theoretical ideas on this list.

Table 8.1   List of Top Mediators

Dimension	**Cognition**	1.	Beliefs
		2.	Cognitive defusion
		3.	Cognitive reappraisal
	Affect	1.	Acceptance
		2.	Anxiety sensitivity
		3.	Self-compassion
	Attention	1.	Mindfulness
		2.	Rumination and worry
		3.	Acting with awareness
	Self	1.	Self-efficacy
		2.	Self-regulation
		3.	Religiousness/spirituality
	Motivation	1.	Values
		2.	Intensions
		3.	Goals
	Behavior	1.	Coping skills
		2.	Behavioral activation
		3.	Avoidance
Level	**Biophysiological**	1.	Neurophysiological
		2.	Dietary intake
		3.	Exercise
	Sociocultural	1.	Parenting
		2.	Social support
		3.	Therapeutic alliance

You can use this table as a reference guide to help you determine how to intervene when a client is stuck in a particular domain. If you wish to choose a focus that is not represented in this table, feel free to do so. As we previously mentioned, this table is not yet final, nor is it exhaustive. You can view this table as a helpful guide containing suggestions, rather than as a rigid book of strict rules.

When we look at Julie's network model, it becomes clear that her struggle falls primarily in the domain of behavior, where she struggles to stand up for herself, avoids difficult conversations, and frequently engages in people pleasing. In table 8.1, we can see that coping skills, avoidance, and behavioral activation are the top three most frequently found behavioral mediators of change.

In Julie's case, overt avoidance seems to play a particularly strong role since she struggles to engage in social contexts that could threaten her sense of self as a nice girl. Going forward, the therapist would be well advised to monitor the extent to which Julie engages in avoidant behavior, which is exactly what happens in the subsequent therapy session.

Therapist: I've been looking at the data in your thought recording and it shows a powerful relationship.

Julie: What did you find?

Therapist: If you are with someone and you have had a thought "I'm selfish" or one of its variants, you are much more likely to then not talk about anything of importance. You are five times more likely not to be talking about *negative* things that are important, which you might expect based on what you told me. But look at this. When you have that "I'm selfish" thought, you are twice as likely to then not talk about *positive* things as compared to when you did not have that thought. It's like that thought is a dimmer switch that keeps intimate conversations away, bad *or* good.

Julie: I knew about the bad, but I'm shocked about the good. I have to think about that. What would that be? What am I doing?

Therapist: I'm not sure, but since "good" conversations are more surprising, let's start there. I think we need more information. I think we need to be more conscious of when that is happening, and how often it happens.

Julie: I'm game.

Therapist: Can you think of a conversation that you would like to have with your husband that is "positive" but that you might avoid and that might somehow be linked to "I'm selfish"?

Julie: (*Pauses*) This is weird, but I can see how this could happen. He's very helpful in playing with the kids when I get home and I'm exhausted. It's so sweet and I notice it and I never actually talk about it. (*Tearing up*) It actually brings tears to my eyes. He's a good guy. I know you probably judged him because he doesn't want me to go to the conference…but it can't just be that he thinks I'm selfish to want to go. He's never said that. He kind of says the opposite (like when he says I'm a people pleaser). But if I notice that he's doing a good job with the kids, I feel guilty and then there go those thoughts again too: *I'm selfish*. I do need to stand up for myself, I do, but I think sometimes I just have a hard time even *being* myself—even when good things are there to be said.

Therapist: Could I ask this of you? Could you deliberately seek out at least two positive conversations with your husband in the next week? Especially try to pick topics that have this unexpected link to "I'm selfish" in your mind. Like you could deliberately thank him for taking good care of the kids. Do your best to have the conversation while staying as open as you can—sort of like being a "mind detective." Then immediately afterward simply journal about it for ten minutes are so…just write about what came up. Then we'll discuss that next session.

Julie: Okay. I'm in.

    This is a kind of behavioral exposure intervention. At this point the target remains Julie's struggle to stand up for herself, but it may be morphing into how to be more genuine—how to be a truer version of Julie. By journaling about a behavioral exposure exercise that undermines her avoidance, Julie and the therapist will have a chance to be more conscious of the functions of her avoidance, shining the spotlight on her automatic habits and better enabling her to actively choose who and how she wants to be in her relationship. Note that for the first time she is actually uncertain about why her husband does not want her to go to the conference—that conversation has not yet been had. If the positive conversations land well, having a more difficult conversation like that will be on the horizon. If we add "Journal about positive conversations with husband" as a new node (and its relations) in Julie's network model, placing it in the behavior dimension of the grid, it will look similar to what we see in figure 8.5.

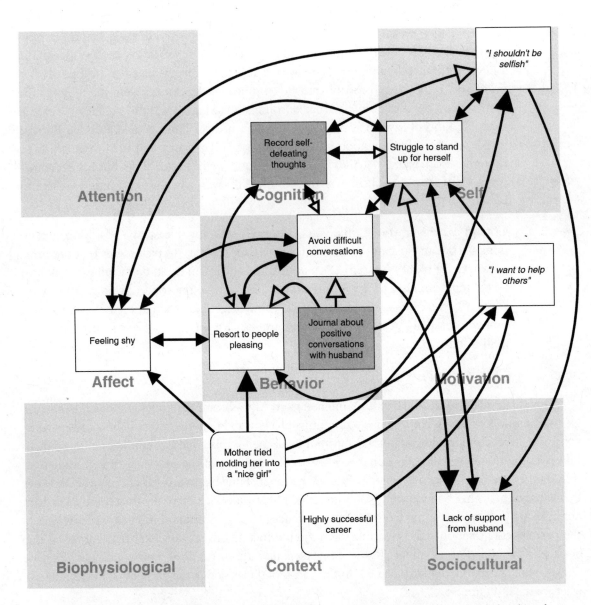

Figure 8.5 Effect of Julie's journaling about positive conversations with husband

Julie has agreed to record the impact of exposure to two positive and intimate conversations with her husband in a previously avoided area that evokes thoughts of selfishness. Note that none of the interventions directly address her feelings of shyness. Although unpleasant and further fueling maladaptive processes, these feelings are only of secondary concern. By targeting Julie's behavior, thoughts, and self-perception, her tendency to feel timid around others is likely going to adjust as a result as well—slowly, but steadily. We have now introduced an additional element to Julie's network model that is supported by existing nodes while weakening existing maladaptive structures. In a subsequent therapy session, Julie will report on what transpired, and, based on her feedback, the therapist and Julie could then decide to take the intervention to the next level (presumably expanding the behavioral exposure exercise) or shift gears to try something entirely different. After all, this was just one approach, and there are many different routes available.

Ultimately, process-based work is always organized around the client's goals. Although we might have our own thoughts about what's best for the client, ultimately, the client decides what is important and what outcomes they hope to achieve. Oftentimes, the initial goal of the client is getting rid of struggles—whether it's depression, anxiety, addiction, or something else entirely. When processes of change are the focus, it is very common for the therapist and client to create a new vision for the client. We can't be sure yet, but Julie may be on the road to working on intimacy issues, relationship-building issues, or communication issues. Unwinding the impact of historically produced thoughts about being selfish may ultimately be more important to her own sense of genuineness than to a simple problem of people pleasing.

We do not want the client to return to therapy indefinitely; instead, we want them to become self-sufficient. In order to help the client get to this point, we have to help them shape their network not only in an adaptive way, but in a self-sustaining one as well. This means we shape the client's network model in a way so that established factors feed into adaptive processes, while maladaptive processes get starved of support. That task may be more or less complex—depending on the complexity of the client's situation, their difficulties, and their goals. You can sometimes flip maladaptive processes in a client's network model into adaptive processes in the same dimension and level, but you need to stay alert to how changes in one area of the network may affect changes in different parts of the network. By zooming in on the processes, you can identify the most relevant ones to yield effective change.

Action Step 8.1 · Adaptive Processes

Let's return to the problem you identified in your own life. Based especially on your answers in Action Step 7.1 (the complete maladaptive EEMM), consider the processes in table 8.1, the List of Top Mediators, and insert in the table below adaptive forms of the processes you think you need to strengthen. Briefly note at least one reason why.

	Adaptive Processes I Need to Strengthen (and Why)
Affect	
Cognition	
Attention	
Self	
Motivation	
Overt Behavior	
Biophysiological	
Sociocultural	

Example

	Adaptive Processes I Need to Strengthen (and Why)
Affect	Acceptance. By entering fearful situations without resorting to escape, I can learn to function effectively within them.
Cognition	Beliefs. By establishing new beliefs that it's okay to embarrass myself and to not be liked, I will work less to avoid either.
Attention	Mindfulness. By practicing awareness in the present moment, I can learn to flexibly shift my focus from what's inside to what happens outside.
Self	Self-efficacy. By setting and achieving goals, I can regain trust in my own abilities.
Motivation	Values. By knowing what truly matters to me, I can focus more on taking steps toward this direction, rather than be dictated by fear.
Overt Behavior	Avoidance. By exposing myself more to fearful situations, I can learn to function better within them.
Biophysiological	–
Sociocultural	Social support. By opening up about my difficulties to trusted people, I can learn to let go of my sense of shame around my fear.

CHAPTER 9

Disrupting the System

Fostering significant change can be hard. The kind of problems people need help with changing have almost always been present for some time, and they are supported by relationships among a network of events. Clients generally have multiple problems and multiple features to any given problem. In this book so far, we've seen few problems that are singular and unidimensional—and that likely applies to you as well as you've taken personally focused action steps. Additional positive goals often also sit behind problem presentations, and your hope may be that one day progress will be made there as well.

This is exactly why using the network approach in thinking about the system that has ensnared your client can be so helpful. In that context, you'll need to give thought to how and where to begin. Like a chess player planning moves, understanding the relationships that exist among the many features of the case allows you to pick targets of change in a way that helps maximize the likelihood of success.

CONSIDERING ALTERNATIVES

There is almost never just one possible path forward in a given case. Multiple options are available—each with its own benefits and drawbacks. Agreement about the treatment plan has to involve client choice and informed consent, but, as the practitioner, you need to think strategically and direct your attention toward alternatives that are most likely to be successful.

When considering different paths forward, keep the following criteria in mind: access, centrality, competence, risk, likelihood of change, and strategic positioning. Depending on how various pathways forward rank on these criteria, some paths will be preferred over others. Let's explore these criteria.

Access refers to the ability to work on a given target, as limited by role, situation, and client willingness. Your professional role may not allow you to open the door to certain issues. In some systems of care, some mental health issues cannot be addressed by drug and alcohol counselors but require counselors with a different expertise. A psychologist working in a chronic pain clinic may be unable to focus on exercise regimens or address medication management because other members of the team have that responsibility. Or, you may work in a setting that only allows a limited number of sessions, making it impossible to dig into complex areas. Additionally, the client themself may limit access. You may think that working on, say, a client's trauma history could be key, but the client may say they are not ready to confront that issue.

Centrality refers to the number and strength of relations sustained between the issue, process of change, and parts of the client's life linked to key outcomes. Speaking just in terms of network properties, the number of edges, or arrows, coming into and out of a node in the network is a kind of operational definition of centrality—at the level of processes of change, the number of edges and subnetworks and their linkage to outcomes define the most central processes.

Competence refers to your training and ability to deliver intervention methods that are likely to alter processes of change. You may be excellent in altering cognitive processes and weak in the steps needed to alter affective ones. You may be fine in values work but weak in defusion work. It's important to strengthen aeras of weakness, of course, but it is also important to use your strengths to foster the best outcomes currently possible, or to refer clients elsewhere if they cannot get needed care from you. As you will see in the next chapter, our very definition of "treatment kernels" includes known competencies so that providers can assess which approaches are most likely to be successful in moving relevant processes in a given clinical situation.

Risk refers to the range of possible outcomes and the relative chance of producing iatrogenic effects. Processes with a lower risk are preferred as intervention points over those with a higher risk potential under the Hippocratic goal of at least doing no harm.

Likelihood of change is the inverse of risk: the probability among the range of outcomes of seeing substantial improvement. Some processes are harder to change than others, and moderators may exist that allow those estimates to be adjusted in an evidence-based way by the characteristics of the client and their situation. In general, it's best to pick targets, especially early, that create positive momentum.

A number of factors are related to the likelihood of change. Processes that have been solidified over a longer period of time will be more likely to resist therapeutic interventions. For instance, a person who has made smoking an integral part of their life for the past thirty years will have a harder time quitting than someone who has been smoking for only a few weeks. Additionally, a client who benefits in some shape or form from their struggles might have a harder time taking steps toward change. For instance, a person who is on disability as a result of particular problems and is therefore receiving financial payments may have a harder time changing in those specific areas because taking steps toward betterment might mean losing some or all of this support. The same can be true of social support, cultural issues, prejudice, stigma, and a whole range of similar issue that could make change harder.

Strategic positioning is perhaps the characteristic most often forgotten, but in some ways, it is the most important feature of a process-based approach. Strategic positioning refers to the likelihood that powerful next steps will open up if the hoped-for change occurs in the targeted process and the targeted area. It is rare to have a client experience a single change and then to be "finished." Even if therapy terminates, it's important to have the person now be situated to take the next positive and needed steps.

If your client has participated in the creation of their own network, which is often a good idea, it is often possible for you to discuss with your client the different pathways forward and weigh these criteria in an open fashion. When the client and you are in agreement on which process to tackle, you can move forward to the next phase. This will include a discussion of risks and benefits of particular treatment kernels—the subject of the next chapter.

Before we turn to a case to explore these issues in a more concrete fashion, it is worth taking a moment to warn against a common clinical error. It is dangerous and dehumanizing to enter into this phase of treatment with an option readily available of explaining failure on the basis of "client resistance," "client personality," or other such judgments that are designed to diminish the pain we feel as providers of not yet knowing how to help everyone. It is empirically true that it is harder to achieve success with some clients than others. For example, clients with chronic, multiple problems of higher severity are indeed less likely to be successful than those whose life situation is less chronic or complex. We may not as a field yet know exactly how to address that fact, even though we recognize that it is our job to learn how. You are likely reading this book right now because you take that job seriously, and in that state of mind you are best prepared to contribute to future solutions. It is a dangerous form of practitioner self-soothing to explain the fact that success can elude us by hanging clinical judgments around the client's neck.

That approach is not helpful because it oversimplifies a complex issue and doesn't foster additional viable strategies to help the client progress. It is also not responsible because it deflects attention away from your own ability to respond. Instead, you would be better advised to take a closer look at the client's network and to investigate which events and processes have led the client to revert back to their old ways. It would also be advisable to change the things you can, such as your own therapeutic competence, your ability to do an adequate process-based functional analysis, or your ability to get client buy-in and to motivate change. The fault lies not with the client as a kind of moral failing, but in the strength and complexity of the network of relations that has them ensnared. Understanding and addressing that is our job, and if we do not have the knowledge or skill needed, we need to carry the pain of that very state of affairs and as a community work to solve it.

PROBING THE SYSTEM

Over the following pages, we will demonstrate what these clinical features of "network thinking" can look like in generating an intervention strategy by returning to a client we met in chapter 6. As you may recall, Michael is a successful entrepreneur who struggles with morning fog. Initially, he was solely concerned that it might affect his work performance, but upon closer investigation, a whole array of other problems came to light. Michael does not exercise and he has unhealthy eating habits, which both contribute to his being overweight. Additionally, he experiences sleeping problems and hypertension. Michael has a history of alcohol abuse, and although he has been in recovery for over five years, he can still notice the aftereffects. He grew up in a relatively poor household, from which he gained certain values that he still holds onto very tightly to this day. Although these values have enabled him to build a successful business, they now seem to stand in the way of his taking better care of his health. In figure 9.1, you can see Michael's network model.

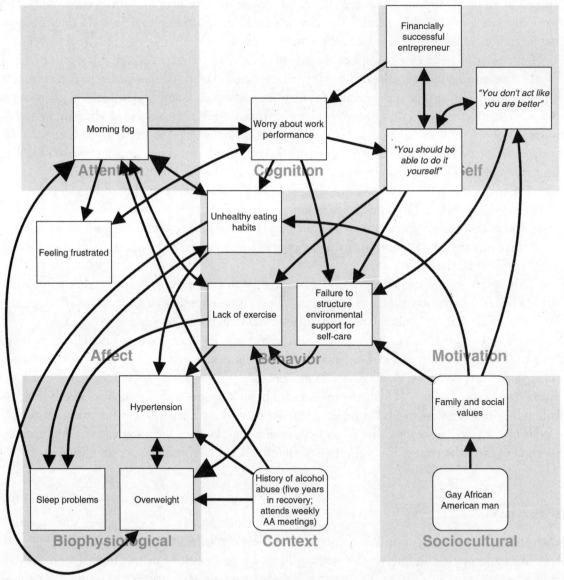

Figure 9.1 Revisiting Michael's network model

Michael's case is quite complex, and you can sense that it may be difficult for him to change because features and processes are strengthened by an array of other features and processes. Affecting change in any node in his network might be hard because almost any relevant process is reinforced from multiple sides. Furthermore, Michael seems to be steadfast in his manner of doing things—after all, it led him to become financially successful in the first place. Central to his clinical situation is the idea that "you should be able to do it by yourself" and that "you don't act like you are better." In conversation with Michael, it became apparent that he holds firmly to these beliefs, which enabled him to build a successful business but which also now stand in his way of accepting outside help.

If the therapist decides to focus on self-care and exercise, these cognitive issues will become central. But given Michael's firm views, creating more cognitive flexibility in this area—either by directly challenging the cognitive system itself or by indirectly doing so (e.g., through defusion work)—might be hard because these ideas have paid off so handsomely in his business. Self-care and exercise could be a good focus if that issue could be addressed, however, because exercise is related not just to his obesity but also to his morning fog and, through that, to his work-related worry.

An alternative pathway could be to try to diminish work-related worry directly in the hopes that it would diminish unhealthy eating habits. However, these habits are also in part cultural, and the clinician may feel that there is even less access there in the sense that Michael may be less willing to attend to that culturally laden issue of food preference than he would be to exercise. That could especially be the case if the therapist is white. Furthermore, exercise is even *more* related to his obesity issues and is just as related to his sleep issues. Conversely, changing his work-related worry in order to change his unhealthy eating habits will not impact his exercise.

Focusing on sleep directly is another possibility, but it might be resistant to change if exercise and diet remain the same. Also, there may be concerns that Michael will want to address sleep first by using sleep medications, which would carry greater downside risks than exercise.

Thus, it's the therapist's task to diminish the influence of Michael's beliefs on matters of his physical health, self-care, and exercise. He may be able to progress the most by working with fitness and nutrition experts. Before that can happen, however, Michael needs to be willing to accept outside help when it comes to his health. He has accepted the help of a psychologist (or else he wouldn't be in therapy), and, as a business owner, he is familiar with delegating tasks to people other than himself. Thinking in terms of processes that would promote greater cognitive flexibility could lead to a different kind of conversation with Michael that creates a cognitive flexibility intervention "on the fly."

MICHAEL'S SELF-CARE

Therapist: I imagine it takes a considerable amount of careful planning and execution to run a business like yours.

Michael: Yes, that would be fair to say.

Therapist: And I assume you often have to delegate tasks to your employees, and rely on their strengths and expertise to do jobs that you wouldn't have the time or the necessary skill for, is that right?

Michael: Yes, definitely. Where are you going with this?

Therapist: I got the impression that when it comes to your business you seem to be very resourceful, and don't hesitate to accept help from others. However, when it comes to your own health, you seem to insist more on fixing things yourself.

Michael: I never thought about it in that way.

Therapist: I wonder if we can take the approach that you so successfully implement at work, and look at your health problems through the same lens?

Michael: You mean getting someone to help me out?

Therapist: For example, yes. In certain ways, this is what we are already doing here in therapy, because you come to these therapy sessions so I can help you get a better grip on your morning fog, right? What if we take this same approach to work on things like your physical fitness or your eating habits?

Michael: I see what you mean. If I'm honest, though, it still seems unnecessary and a bit pompous to me. I mean me get a "trainer"? La de dah.

Therapist: I get it. And yet it seems that you have been dealing with these issues for some time now by yourself, is that right? So if you would continue doing what you have done before, what does your experience tell you how this will work?

Michael: Well, I probably get the same results *(chuckles)*.

Therapist: I think so too. But you know, accepting outside help does not necessarily require an expensive fitness trainer. There's a fitness center open 24/7 very near you and it's not pricey. They have classes all the time that are free for members. Or you could even just join a workout group, or start exercising with a friend. But you are not an island—there's no reason not to bring your "business mind" to this challenge.

Michael: Funny, I've noticed that health club and I've thought about joining multiple times. I even have friends who go there! But almost instantly I then think, *Just do it yourself,* and the chain of thinking ends. But you are right about this: I don't do that in my business. If I really need help, I get what help I need. I'd have failed ten times over if I hadn't done that.

Therapist: You don't have to commit to anything just yet if you don't feel ready, but I would like to ask you to really think about which steps you would start taking if you would approach your health more as you do a business problem. What would you do differently?

In this conversation segment, the therapist opened up to Michael the idea to approach his health issues like a business problem. This is a *cognitive reframing* intervention, the details of which were created in the moment, by finding an overarching thought that would better support new ways of thinking about his situation. Since Michael is used to delegating tasks to third parties and seeks out help when it comes to issues of his business, he might feel more inclined to do the same when it comes to his own health if his situation is framed that way.

Seeing how this reframe immediately loosens up Michael's approach, the therapist quickly tags and restates that "reframe" at the end of the conversation and then gives a small bit of homework so as to nail it down: to "really think about which steps you would start taking if you would approach your health as a business problem."

This approach works around the cognitive inflexibility that comes from adherence to the beliefs that "you should be able to do it yourself" and "you don't act like you are better." The therapist has not challenged these beliefs or diminished them—instead he has linked self-care to well-established verbal rules that are familiar and successful. If we add the new node "Approach health problems like business problems" (and its relations) to Michael's network model, it will look like figure 9.2.

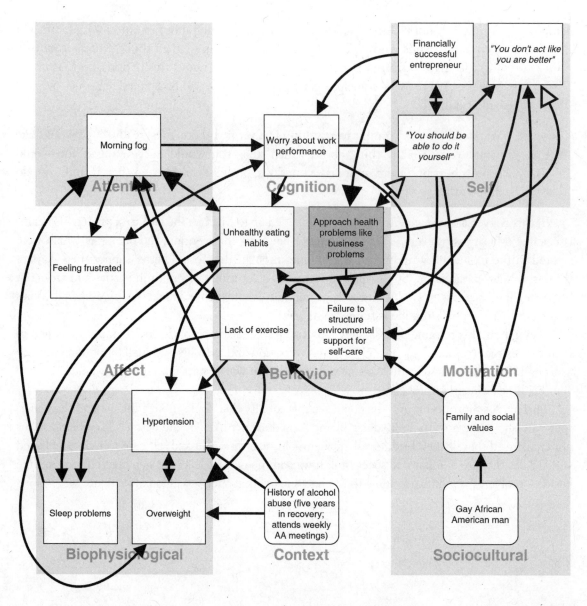

Figure 9.2 Reframing a new approach for Michael

As you can see, this simple idea can already diminish the effect of Michael's strict beliefs, which otherwise would make him resist interventions. In return, this new approach is fueled by Michael's experience as a successful entrepreneur, and in some ways even by his pattern of "doing things by himself," since he drew from that conviction to build his business in the first place.

Note that this intervention alone changes nothing about Michael's core concerns—his morning fog, sleeping problems, and worry about his work performance—but it sets up concrete steps that Michael can take to implement the idea of approaching his health problems in a similar way to how he would approach problems in his business. After this intervention, Michael joins the health club and begins taking classes. He likes them but soon discovers he will work even harder with a personal trainer who works there. Some of his friends use the trainer as well, and he soon finds that it simply feels responsible and supportive, not like "acting like you are better." All of his health measures improve (overweight, sleep, morning fog, hypertension), but he still has a ways to go. This all can be shown in the next network (figure 9.3). If we add the new node "Workout with personal trainer" (and its relations) to Michael's network model, it will look like figure 9.3.

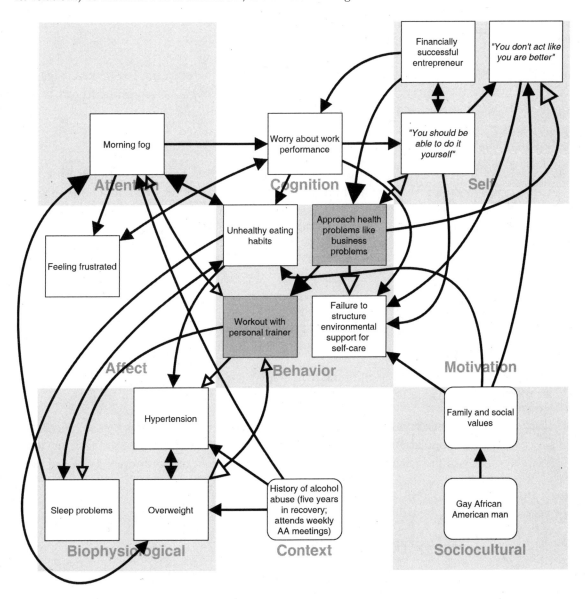

Figure 9.3 Effect of Michael's workout with a personal trainer

There are two ways forward with Michael at this point. There is still the option of working directly on his work-related worry. It's lessened because the morning fog has improved, but the main reason to go there might be to get additional leverage on his unhealthy eating habits.

The main alternative to that strategy is to work on the eating habits directly. This will be challenging because it's a family cultural pattern, but Michael already has made gains altering another cultural pattern, namely the beliefs that "you should be able to do it yourself" and "you don't act like you are better," by reframing needed steps as an extension of his business acumen.

In discussion with Michael, the therapist puts that "business of living" challenge in front of him.

Therapist: You've made a lot of progress.

Michael: I have. Really, I have. I feel better than I have in many years. I still need to get my blood pressure and weight down, and the sleep problems and morning fog are still an issue I guess, but I've made so much progress.

Therapist: What's your doctor say is the main issue now?

Michael: Well, she says I won't get to where I need to be unless I change how I'm eating. Way too much fat. Way too much meat. But that's what I know; it's how I cook; it's how my family cooked. That's home cooking in my world. I mean actually I even *like* healthy food. I like salads. I like fish. I like vegetables. I just don't eat it. I don't even know how to make most of that.

Therapist: And so…

Michael: Don't even look at me like that! (*smiling*) I know what you are thinking. Look, a trainer is one thing…but I'm not getting a cook! I mean I could afford it, but damn… that's just not me. My mother would roll over in her grave.

Therapist: Okay. I admit it. I was thinking that! But what else? Bring your "my health is my business" mindset to it.

Michael: Well, I don't know… Maybe this. I saw an ad on TV for one of those things that became popular during the COVID era: "We will bring healthy food to your door." That was the pitch. There were fliers for it at the health club even. It looked good actually.

Therapist: Would you be willing to give that a go?

Michael: Why not? Nothing done, nothing won.

By suggesting that Michael approach his health as he approaches his business, the therapist was able to revise the network as shown in figure 9.4. The healthy meal-plan subscription shows a positive influence on his morning fog, hypertension, sleep, and weight problems. It's an effective intervention for targeting some key health issues.

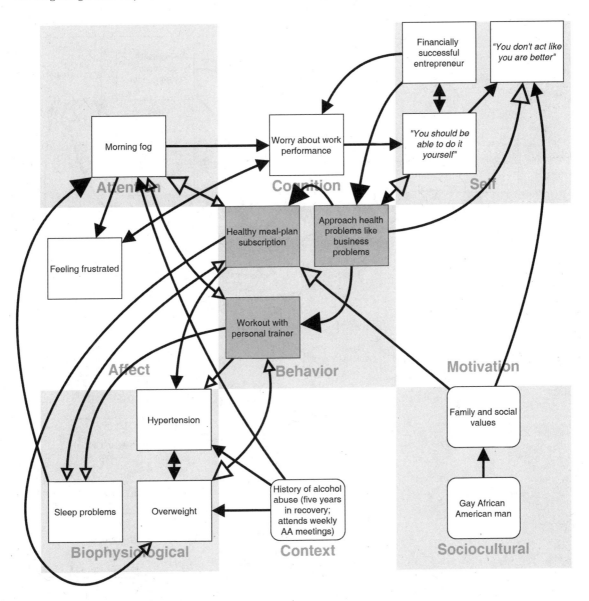

Figure 9.4 Effect of Michael's healthy meal-plan subscription

SIMPLIFYING THE NETWORK

If Michael could make continued progress, the problem nodes in the area of health would begin to fall out of the network. If they all reach a reasonable level, the network would become considerably more simple. This is shown in figure 9.5.

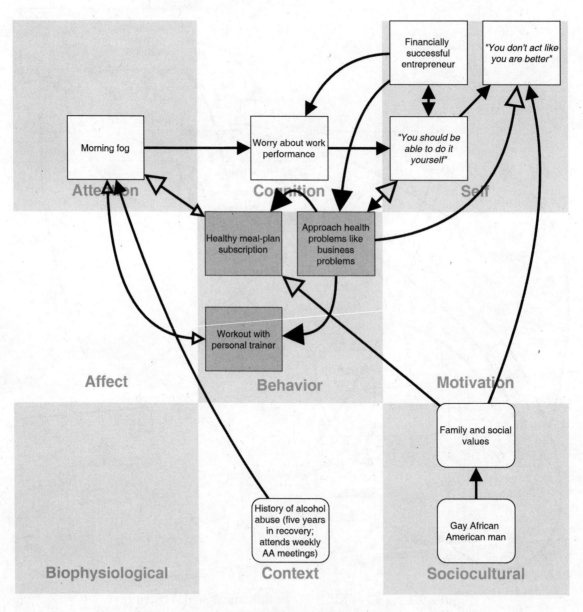

Figure 9.5 Michael's case resolution

Michael still worries about work, but not at a level that he sees as a problem. Morning fog is still a minor issue, an echo of his years of alcohol abuse, but he successfully manages the health problems he can by bringing his full set of business management skills to the table...and the gym. Instead of being a barrier to his health, his family values of independence, humility, and hard work are now supporting his self-care and health by being an extension of his approach to challenges as a successful business manager.

The key process of change in this case was greater cognitive flexibility as established by reframing health challenges hierarchically within his mental approach to business success. That reframe avoided the direct cognitive conflict that was keeping him from adjusting to these health challenges in new ways, and allowed his competence in problem solving to come to the fore. The entry target chosen was mindful of the ease of access, centrality, competence, risk, likelihood of change, and strategic positioning issues of the various alternatives so that the likelihood of successfully disrupting the system was maximized.

LOOKING OUT FOR TIPPING POINTS

A change in the network can sometimes happen quite suddenly. In fact, therapeutic change is rarely a slow and continuous process. Much more commonly, the system shows only very little initial change, despite considerable effort by the client and therapist. This is because a complex network is very resilient to outside pressure. When the change finally happens, it happens abruptly once the network reaches a tipping point. Such a change in the stability of a network can be depicted with a ball rolling from one valley (position 1) over a hill (position 2) to another valley (position 3). (figure 9.6).

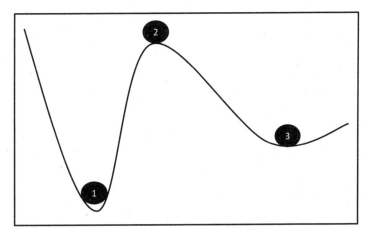

Figure 9.6 Tipping point of a dynamic system.

A network is more resilient and stable if the valley is deep (as in position 1) because it requires more effort to move the ball out of the valley and over the hill. But once the ball reaches the tipping point (position 2), a sudden shift can occur even after a small additional perturbation. As a result, the network undergoes a dramatic shift, leading to a new alternative and stable state (position 3).

Depending on a number of factors, this new state may be more or less resistant to change. The example in figure 9.6 shows that the new network structure is relatively less resistant to change because the valley is relatively shallow (position 3) and less effort is required to move the ball out of the valley. Obviously, this would be good news for Michael, because less effort is necessary to reinstate the adaptive state.

In general, networks comprising highly interconnected nodes can reach such a tipping point when a local perturbation causes a domino effect, cascading into a systemic transition after outside disturbances reach a critical threshold. In contrast, networks that are not highly interconnected (i.e., networks characterized by weakly or incompletely connected elements) are more likely to change more gradually in response to such perturbations.

One common condition for reaching a transition point is a positive feedback loop that, once a critical point is reached, propels the system to change toward an alternate state. Two features are important for the overall response of such systems: first, the heterogeneity of the nodes, and second, their connectivity. The reason for this is that the connectivity and homogeneity of the network determine the stability of network.

Virtually all complex networks have in common these generic features we have been discussing. These features can be important markers of the fragility that typically precedes abrupt changes that might signal a critical transition that could lead to a tipping point. This could be of great value for mental health because mathematical models of such networks could predict the remission of a disorder, and it may provide a critical window for early intervention to prevent relapse or even the onset of a problem.

Although it is outside the scope of this book, digital mental health technology is coming to PBT work. It will soon allow practitioners to gather ecological momentary assessment data to inform the dynamic network of a client, which will indicate the presence of any tipping points that might precede clinically significant events. Already there are indications that idiographic complex network analysis can do a better job of predicting important events, such as treatment dropout, treatment gains, the onset of panic attacks, manic episodes, psychotic breaks, and even suicidality, before these events are evident using other measures and means. But how can we effectively disturb a maladaptive network? What are the specific treatment strategies that we have available as effective clinicians? The next chapter will review some of these strategies. We call them *treatment kernels* because they are the basic elements of intervention strategies designed to modify processes of change.

CHAPTER 10

Treatment Kernels

Humans are complex systems. That is true at the individual level, and it is equally true of the complex social systems they form. Psychotherapy is a dynamic process that is intended to bring about adaptive change in these complex systems. Processes of change are functional sequences, not mere snapshots. If change processes are to serve as part of an alternative to the DSM/ICD, then these processes must directly and successfully lead to the selection and implementation of intervention strategies. The basic elements of these strategies are *treatment kernels*—specific change methods designed to modify processes of change. We will discuss and illustrate some of those kernels in this chapter.

Although evidence-based intervention began in a process-focused direction, over the last forty years it has become synonymous with treatment protocols for specific psychiatric syndromes as defined by the DSM and ICD. It has become agonizingly clear that this approach is limited in terms of both efficacy and clinical utility. Clients never nominated "symptoms" to be the focus of their lives—that came from the well-meaning biomedicalization of human suffering and the gradual cultural change that conception produced. After receiving evidence-based intervention, a relatively large number of patients remain "symptomatic," and a larger percentage feel that their problems (which often extended beyond classic syndromal signs and symptoms in the first place) were not fully and adequately addressed. On the treatment-delivery side of the equation, it is neither feasible nor meaningful to train clinicians in all of the so-called evidence-based treatment protocols, many of which take many months of training to climb over the hurdles constructed by treatment developers.

When all of these issues are combined, the result is grim: too few clients receive an evidence-based treatment that plausibly targets their specific problems; too few reach a fully satisfactory end state; and too few clinicians are adequately trained to deliver these needed evidence-based treatments. Meanwhile, as a systems matter, the prevalence of psychological problems is rising, not falling.

A positive intermediate step has been the development of modular treatments. Instead of entire treatment protocols for specific DSM- or ICD-defined disorders, some clinical researchers have examined the utility of a smaller number of treatment components that can be used or left on the shelf as needed. Even in these early stages, there is evidence that a modular approach is more efficient and effective than a protocol-for-syndrome approach (e.g., Weisz et al., 2012). Often these modules target specific problems, such as behavioral modules designed to reinforce prosocial behavior and to discourage aggressive behaviors in children with conduct disorder. Other clinical researchers have created modular interventions that apply to many problem areas with a small set of component interventions. These include the so called "transdiagnostic" interventions such as the unified protocol (Barlow et al., 2010) and ACT (Hayes et al., 2016).

A logical next step in this approach is to identify the key elements that constitute treatment modules and to determine how they engage processes of change. With that knowledge in hand, it becomes possible for intervention to involve the person-specific identification and competent delivery of treatment kernels that are likely to modify idiographically relevant processes of change.

We believe that some of the needed evidence to take that next step is already in hand, for example, in known processes of change linked to existing component analyses, or in the creation and use of a variety of more limited protocols, such as those in web, app, book, and telephone-based protocols. Other examples of evidence are process and outcome changes from very short (e.g., single-session) protocols. As PBT sensibilities impact our research, more idiographic longitudinal complex network data are also becoming available.

The process-based vision is that theoretically and empirically coherent sets of change processes can be applied to a wide array of problem domains in an individually tailored manner—presenting practitioners with a far less daunting training task of how to use change processes to fit treatment kernels to client needs. While well-crafted and empirically supported models of change processes are needed, this approach does not require treatment methods to be linked to an *a priori* commitment to broad "schools" or to comprehensive "one size fits all" protocols. In fact, our hope is that PBT can accommodate any treatment kernel that is empirically based and properly linked to evidence-based processes of change, thereby making technologically defined packages and "therapy schools" obsolete.

Metaphorically, treatment kernels can be thought of as construction elements. If someone is building a house, they might need bricks and windows, sinks and faucets, doors and lumber. It would be odd to limit these elements to a particular brand: the best windows might be made by one company and the best doors by another. That being said, it matters whether you are building a house or a garden shed, so the utility of any particular construction element has to be seen in terms of the purpose and stage of the construction.

In the same way, practitioners need to use what is needed for the individual client to construct an intervention approach that is likely to get the job done. At the level of treatment kernels or techniques, functional eclecticism makes sense, but not in an empty or mindless way. In a PBT approach, treatment kernels are there to accomplish an empirically and conceptually necessary task: to engage and alter specific processes of change.

When we focus on which processes need to be altered and how, which has been the focus of this book up until now, a more manageable set of choices emerges. Processes are hierarchically arranged—some are broad and multifaceted, such as psychological flexibility, whereas others are more elementary, such as reinforcing habit change. The same is true of treatment kernels. Some intervention modules, such as contemplative practice, are known to change several important processes of change. Others, such as relaxation training, are more focused on particular rows of the EEMM.

We are not able yet to give a comprehensive list of treatment kernels. That is true in part due to the hegemony of the "protocols-for-syndromes" era. So much research effort was focused on overall treatment protocols that component analyses were chronically given short shrift in many wings of evidence-based therapy. In addition, a syndromal focus so undermined attention to processes of change that kernels were not systematically linked empirically to change processes. In other words, the limitations of the "protocols-for-syndromes" era are still with us as the era of PBT unfolds.

Fortunately, this picture is changing rapidly. Meta-analyses of components linked to processes are beginning to appear (e.g., Levin et al., 2012), suggesting that an empirically derived list of treatment kernels might be possible sometime in the future beyond our initial and limited attempt (Hayes & Hofmann, 2018). In this chapter we will only give examples, and we acknowledge that kernels are overlapping and differ in level of specificity such that some kernels might be conceived of as a combination or modification of other kernels.

We can give the following working definition of treatment kernels: these are *functionally organized and empirically supported classes of intervention methods that are tied to a reasonably comprehensive and testable theoretical model, that are known to impact particular evidence-based processes of change and subsequent outcomes as a result, and that are sufficiently well specified technologically to provide known therapeutic competencies for their acquisition and delivery.* Stated less formally, treatment kernels are sets of specified methods that when learned and deployed have been shown to move particular processes of change and subsequent outcomes in a predictable fashion.

Let's use our construction metaphor to explain what we mean. If you need to let in natural light when building a house, you need a window or skylight. Bricks or sinks will simply never do the job. There may be a wide range of windows and skylights available in a wide range of sizes, shapes, colors, and materials. Some are better than others for given applications. A good builder needs to master the installation of enough of these to meet consumer needs and perhaps even to know how to create a window from scratch for a special purpose. Knowing how to install a single size and type of window will simply not do.

Similarly, every clinician should be familiar with a sufficient range of treatment kernels in order to be effective when working within reasonably well supported and comprehensive models of analysis and interventions. By "reasonably comprehensive," we mean that the model covers enough of the issues noted in the EEMM to be a good and flexible guide to analysis and intervention. The most effective clinician will be the one who is able to combine these kernels in such a way that they optimally target the crucial processes in a given client in the given context. This is the foundation of PBT.

One implication of thinking of kernels as a functional class is that some kernels might need to be created in vivo to fit the client's idiosyncratic need. If kernels are created "on the fly," they can rapidly become evidence based to a certain extent by careful specification of their proximal process targets for the individual clients and their theoretical links to kernels of known impact. Part of the beauty of PBT as a model of evidence-based practice is that it both embraces and channels clinical creativity. As long as a process of change is well established empirically and is clearly of relevance to the client, any method that moves these processes in a positive direction can be thought of as part of an evidence-based approach.

We described a number of treatment kernels in our book *Process-Based CBT* (Hayes & Hofmann, 2018). These were based on the consensus results of the Interorganizational Task Force on Cognitive and Behavioral Psychology Doctoral Education (Klepac et al., 2012). The charge of this task force was to identify core competencies to develop guidelines for integrating doctoral education and training in cognitive and behavioral psychology in the United States. The task force (Klepac et al., 2012) listed a set of core clinical competencies that we later expanded and elaborated upon (Hayes & Hofmann, 2018). We will review a few of them here briefly, but we encourage you to consult our earlier text for a more detailed discussion and illustration of these competencies and kernels. Still, it has to be acknowledged that as a field we are still "feeling our way." Some of the kernels noted by the task force are still too broad; some are more processes of change than kernels; and additional ones exist. Let's begin to examine a few.

SOME KERNELS TARGETING ATTENTION

We commonly focus on things in our environment that are of importance and pay less attention to things that are not overly important. Said in a more technical way, by our actions we can augment or diminish the stimulus control exerted over our psychological actions by internal or external events.

The act of attending is a cognitive action and, like all psychological events, is a limited resource. There are only so many seconds in a day, and there are only so many things one can notice or attend to. We can sense the limitations of this resource when attempting to split our attention between two or more things. In many situations, multitasking has a cost for all of the actions we are trying to combine. This is why texting while driving is often deadly.

This is not to say that we can't jump and chew gum at the same time. We can do so to some extent, as long as both tasks are fairly automatic and require little additional cognitive management. Texting is not automatized and thereby requires significant cognitive and attentional resources; to some degree driving is automatized but not in a way that can respond quickly and safely to complexity or to the unexpected. It is not only texting behavior that interferes with driving; even talking to somebody hands-free while driving increases the risk of an accident because our attention is captured by a task other than driving.

We pay attention to things that are of importance and we ignore or automatize other things. Obviously, the same thing can be important for one person but not very important at all or even unimportant for another person. A dog owner and dog lover will pay a lot more attention to the dogs in her neighborhood than somebody who cares not at all about pets; an ornithologist will pay a lot more attention to birds than somebody who doesn't care about birds.

Our experience and attitudes shape our attention. If you grow up in a country with a lot of insects and spiders, you are unlikely to be afraid of those types of insects and spiders. In fact, tarantulas are considered a delicacy in some native cultures. If you grow up in such a culture, you will have a very different relationship to tarantulas than if you have never interacted with a tarantula before. Conversely, many people with excessive fear of spiders avoid even looking at spiders. Sometimes, their fear decreases when they are encouraged to repeatedly look at spider pictures.

An example of an attention kernel is based on this observation. Researchers have developed a computerized training procedure that has become known as *attention bias modification* (see Beard et al., 2012 for a meta-analysis). It is an example of a relatively narrowly focused treatment kernel. This training procedure is based on the fact that simply repeatedly presenting spider pictures—even subliminally (i.e., presenting the picture so briefly that the person is not aware of having seen the picture)—can lead to a reduction in fear for some people.

This is not only true for spiders, of course. Maladaptive self-focused attention is a key feature of social anxiety for many people struggling with performance anxiety. When confronted with a social threat, such as while delivering a public speech, some people with social anxiety focus their attention on themselves and their internal events rather than on the topic they are discussing and how best to serve their audience. As a result, it can be hard to attend to their own argument and whether important points are being adequately covered or stated clearly—key cognitive tasks for a successful speech performance. Instead, they focus on themselves, sometimes even feeling like they are looking at themselves. As they sense they are losing focus on the task at hand, their fears may increase further. If they double down and pay even more attention to themselves— their body, their heart racing, blushing, and so on—they may lose the thread of their talk entirely.

The same vicious cycle can be seen in some people with erectile dysfunction: rather than augmenting the impact of sexual cues, they might focus on their anxiety and performance—events that are not intrinsically sexually arousing. Attentional processes are the initial cognitive stages that are often linked to fears around social performance. *Attention training procedures* allow the person to allocate attention in a more flexible, fluid, and voluntary way. One quite common strategy to modify attentional processes is *mindfulness training*.

Mindfulness is a component of many of the newer behavior therapies (mindfulness-based stress reduction, acceptance and commitment therapy, dialectical behavior therapy, mindfulness-based cognitive therapy, and others). Mindfulness is a broad term with many different varieties, but virtually all forms include attentional training. Vipassana-style methods that involve "following the breath," for example, allow the person to notice when attention wanders and to bring it back to the breath as a focus. Mindfulness methods help free individuals from a habitual focus on the past and future—the source of rumination and worry—and anchor their awareness in the present moment. In essence, mindfulness processes initiate attention reallocation, from future threats or past losses and failures to present-moment sensory experience, and from cognitive processes to specific sensations.

Mindfulness practices include body scan meditation, breath counting meditation, mindfulness in daily life, and loving-kindness and compassion meditation, among many others. We will not summarize them here and instead refer the reader to our text (Hayes & Hofmann, 2018) and other sources.

Mindfulness raises an important issue that we need to note with regard to our "functional class" definition of kernels. Most mindfulness practices engage a number of different processes of change. Learning to pay attention in this way requires some degree of emotion regulation, cognitive openness, and detachment from a self-narrative. This breadth does not cancel its usefulness as a kernel. There is no a priori reason for all kernels to target one and only one process of change. Some do, and some don't. It is more important to know which processes are engaged by a given kernel and to know either that all of these processes are of relevance to a particular case or at least that key processes will likely be moved and other process changes will not be interfering. Even simple kernels may engage multiple processes. Social skills training, for example, targets overt behavior but is usually done in a way that is a de facto form of exposure, with resulting affective impact. Thus, while mindfulness may stand out because of it its level of complexity, its broad impact does not disqualify it as a kernel.

SOME KERNELS TARGETING COGNITIONS

Most forms of evidence-based therapy, and certainly those that are part of the behavioral and cognitive therapies, include many kernels targeting cognitions. One of the most popular models that structures the use of processes and kernels is the CBT model develop by Aaron Beck (1976) and colleagues. In this approach, alterations in thinking styles, such as automatic thoughts and cognitive schemata, are argued to account for therapeutic benefits. This treatment approach is thus directed toward modifying the client's maladaptive beliefs and deactivating them while making other schemata available. Thoughts are considered hypotheses that are expressed in the form of automatic thoughts in a given situation or overarching beliefs about oneself, the future, or the world.

Before looking at examples of how Beck's model links processes of cognitive change to treatment kernels, it is worth noticing that models are currently necessary to make full use of a process-based approach. The EEMM is a model of models—it is not a model in itself. Knowing that cognition is important, and that cognitive rigidity can be unhelpful, is not alone enough to intervene in this dimension. To help make this point we will describe cognitive processes from Beck's (1976) model along with cognitive kernels that target them, and then briefly examine a process drawn from a newer form of behavioral and cognitive therapy and kernels it suggests.

The central notion of Beck's model is simple. It is the idea that our behavioral and emotional responses are strongly influenced by our cognitions (i.e., thoughts), which determine how we perceive things. That is, we are only anxious, angry, or sad if we think that we have reason to be anxious, angry, or sad. In other words, it is not the situation per se, but rather our perceptions, expectations, and interpretations (i.e., the cognitive appraisal) of events that are responsible for our emotions (see Hofmann, 2011 for more details). This might be best illustrated to a client by using the following classic example provided by Beck (1976):

The Essence of the Cognitive Approach

("The housewife," Beck, 1976, pp. 234–235)

A [woman] hears a door slam. Several hypotheses occur to her: "It may be Sally returning from school." "It might be a burglar." "It might be the wind that blew the door shut." The favored hypothesis should depend on her taking into account all the relevant circumstances. The logical process of hypothesis testing may be disrupted, however, by the housewife's psychological set. If her thinking is dominated by the concept of danger, she might jump to the conclusion that it is a burglar. She makes an arbitrary inference. Although such an inference is not necessarily incorrect, it is based primarily on internal cognitive processes rather than actual information. If she then runs and hides, she postpones or forfeits the opportunity to disprove (or confirm) the hypothesis.

This example could be used as a discussion point with the client to illustrate that the same event (hearing the slamming of the door) elicits very different emotions depending on how the person interprets the situational context. The door slam itself does not elicit any emotions one way or the other. But when we believe that the door slam suggests that there is a burglar in the house, we may experience fear. We might jump to this conclusion more readily if we are somehow primed after having read about burglaries in the paper, or if our core belief (schema) is that the world is dangerous place and that it is only a matter of time until a burglar will enter our house. Our behavior, of course, would be very different if we felt than the event had no significant meaning.

By treating thoughts as hypotheses that may contain cognitive errors, clients are put into the role of observers or scientists rather than passive victims of psychological problems. Some problems might be fostered by *probability overestimation,* the belief that an unlikely event is likely to happen. Others may be based on *catastrophic thinking,* in which the negative impact of possible outcomes is blown out of proportion.

Examples of treatment kernels that may target these cognitive errors would be using information from patients' past experiences to note how realistic or unrealistic probability estimates may be (e.g., "What is the likelihood based on your past experience?"); delivering more accurate information through psychoeducation (e.g., "Here is what is known about the chance that panic will lead to a sudden heart attack"); using Socratic questioning to help reevaluate the outcome of a situation (e.g., "What is the worst thing that could happen?"); and giving clients behavioral tests to evaluate their hypotheses in vivo by exposing them to feared or avoided activities and situations (e.g., "Let see if it is true that you can no longer do anything worthwhile for your family. What might you want to try to do tomorrow that might be helpful?"). Finally, *cognitive reappraisal methods* would be used to encourage alternative ways to think about the event, such as by asking clients, "What are alternative ways of interpreting this particular event?" or "How would other people interpret this event?" and using self-monitoring forms to guide this process.

Newer forms of behavioral and cognitive therapy, such as ACT, conceptualize cognitive inflexibility in a somewhat different way. ACT practitioners can apply the psychological flexibility model to the EEMM in a straightforward way because the six flexibility/inflexibility processes comport with the six psychological rows of the EEMM. In the psychological flexibility model underlying ACT, the biggest problem with cognition is that it tends to be too habitual, narrow, and focused on literal truth rather than open, flexible, and focused on workability. One of the key maladaptive processes of change in this approach is cognitive fusion—the tendency for cognition to dominate unnecessarily over other useful sources of behavioral control due to clients' treating thoughts literally or not noticing that thoughts are structuring their world. *Cognitive defusion* is the adaptive process that counteracts fusion, and defusion kernels can be used to reduce that unhelpful automatic domination.

The scores of defusion methods that have been tested are all functionally similar: they alter the context of cognition so as to experience the presence of thoughts in a more open, curious, and self-compassionate way while not allowing them to restrict action unnecessarily. Examples of methods that are part of a defusion kernel include distilling a maladaptive thought down to a single word and saying it rapidly and repeatedly out loud for thirty seconds; saying difficult thoughts aloud in the voice of yourself as a young child; and guided imagery exercises that involve imagining thoughts floating by, written on leaves on a stream. Because kernels are functional classes of methods, a single kernel could contain hundreds of functionally similar alternatives, just as there are hundreds of sizes and types of windows, but all are windows. What selects among them are the details of the case. That process of refinement will become fully empirical only as data are gathered.

We have repeatedly emphasized that PBT opens the door to consideration of all evidence-based processes and kernels, but we have also emphasized that processes must be theoretically coherent. The following two examples show why both of these things are true. First, a traditional CBT clinician taking a process-based approach could use defusion kernels linked to the kind of cognitive distancing that Beck believed was necessary to successfully reappraise habitual cognitive patterns. A defusion kernel might also be used to target *thought-action fusion*—the difficulty of separating cognitions from behaviors (e.g., Hofmann, 2011). It appears that thought-action fusion comprises either the belief that experiencing a particular thought increases the chance that the event will actually occur (likelihood), or the belief that thinking about an action is practically identical to actually performing the action (morality). This moral component is assumed to be the result of the erroneous conclusion that experiencing "bad" thoughts is indicative of one's "true" nature and intentions. For example, the thought of killing another person may be considered morally equivalent to performing the act. In this case, a defusion kernel is being used to target a process that is coherent within the cognitive therapy model.

In the second example, a person working with ACT as a form of process-based therapy could similarly use methods drawn from the cognitive reappraisal kernel (probably after cognitive defusion methods were successfully applied) to help brainstorm a wider range of possible thoughts that could be tested for their workability. In that case reappraisal would not be used to challenge and change existing thoughts but to allow more cognitive and response flexibility in the presence of thoughts that are inducing psychological rigidity.

What would likely not make sense is to mix processes and kernels in a philosophically and conceptually incoherent way, such as using a defusion kernel to challenge thoughts or using reappraisal to promote mindful awareness of thought. PBT is not a call for pouring all treatment methods into a big pot and calling it gumbo. Functionally speaking, kernels target processes of change, and processes of change require theory and models to be properly understood.

SOME KERNELS TARGETING AFFECT

A variety of kernels are particularly associated with targeting affect. A well-known maladaptive emotion regulation strategy is *experiential avoidance* (Hayes, 2004), the attempt to eliminate or diminish the form, frequency, or situational sensitivity of affect even when doing so causes psychological difficulty. An affect-focused kernel linked to experiential avoidance is *acceptance,* taking the time to feel emotion and other experiences and learn from them without needless defense. Acceptance methods include guided exercises in noticing how emotion impacts bodily sensations, memory, behavioral urges, or thoughts; exploring emotion experience in nontypical ways (e.g., if it were a color what color would it be; if it had a shape what shape would it have); learning to let go of needless defenses during emotional imagery; observing and describing the emotional impact of events in a more fine-grained way; and so on. All of these methods can be thought of as a kind of exposure, but in the service of exploring the affective domain, not subtracting from or eliminating it.

Progressive muscular relaxation training is one of the most empirically studied kernels linked to affect. In its classical form it involves deliberately tensing and relaxing specific muscle groups so as to learn the felt difference and to be able to "let go" of muscular tension voluntarily. A wide variety of other deliberate forms of relaxation or emotional regulation have emerged over the years, including guided imagery, forms of meditation, yoga, breathing training, and the like.

The close link between affect and cognition in humans means that many cognitive methods are also used for affective purposes. Emotional suppression, for example, has often been shown to be unhelpful, and characteristically these efforts are supported by unhelpful beliefs. The paradoxical effect of suppression is that the harder we try not to be bothered by something, the more this something is bothering us, whether in the form of feelings, thoughts, images, or events in our surrounding environment (such as a dripping water faucet or the ticking of a clock). This phenomenon may be illustrated in the White Bear Experiment by Dan Wegner (Wegner, 1994).

The White Bear Experiment

(Wegner, 1994)

1. Picture a fluffy, white bear.

2. Think for 1 minute about anything you like, except the fluffy white bear.

3. Every time the white bear pops into your mind, count it by lifting your fingers.

Now consider the following:

- How many white bears popped into your mind? Chances are that the bear popped into you mind a few times. Some people think of it only a few times; others a lot. It is very rare that somebody does not think of it at all.

- Notice that you only thought of the white bear after you were asked not to think of a white bear. The mere attempt not to think of it was the reason why you thought of it.

- How good does it feel to think of a white bear? Chances are that the thought becomes annoying because it is intrusive, similar to a song that you can't get out of your mind.

Wegner found that attempts to suppress thoughts paradoxically increased the frequency of such thoughts during a post-suppression period in which participants were free to think about any topic (Wegner, 1994). The reason why a neutral image of a white bear became an intrusive image was simply because of the attempt to suppress it. The reason for this paradoxical effect is related to the cognitive activity that is required in order to suppress it. In order to not think about something, we have to monitor our cognitive processes. As part of this monitoring process, we focus on the very thing that we are trying not to focus on, which leads to the paradox and, when done regularly, could potentially lead to emotional disorders. Research has indeed shown links between this rebound effect as a laboratory phenomenon and clinical disorders. For example, thought suppression leads to increased electrodermal responses to emotional thoughts (Wegner, 1994), suggesting that it elevates sympathetic arousal. Similarly, ruminating about unpleasant events prolongs both angry and depressed moods, and attempts to suppress pain are similarly unproductive.

Think of what would happen if the image were not a neutral white bear but an emotional event, such as a rape trauma. Personally meaningful or emotionally valanced thoughts or images are notably harder to suppress. Generally speaking, many psychiatric problems are related to ineffective attempts to regulate unwanted experiences, such as feelings, thoughts, and images. Thus, most cognitive treatment kernels (e.g., mindfulness, reappraisal, defusion) can also be deployed for affective purposes.

SOME KERNELS TARGETING MOTIVATION

An example of a motivational kernel is *motivational interviewing*. It can be a highly effective treatment kernel to help initiate behavior change. Although motivational interviewing is widely applicable, it is particularly common in the treatment of addiction. Below, we present an example of this technique in the context of a drinking problem.

Charlie's Drinking Problem

Therapist: Please help me understand some of the reasons why you drink.

Charlie: Well, it makes me feel good. It's a way for me to unwind and kick back with my buddies.

Therapist: So you drink because it's a way to enjoy spending time with your friends.

Charlie: Right.

Therapist: What would happen if you didn't drink when you get together with your friends?

Charlie: It would be pretty weird. I don't think it would be much fun. My friends would think that there is something wrong with me, you know?

Therapist: I understand. So your friends would be surprised because it's part of your friendship.

Charlie: Yes, I guess.

Therapist: What would you do if you did not go out drinking with your friends?

Charlie: That would be pretty boring. I would probably stay home.

Therapist: I see. So staying home is boring, whereas you would have fun going out drinking with your friends.

Charlie: Right. It wouldn't just be boring. It would be bloody depressing.

Therapist: Because you are alone?

Charlie: Yes.

Therapist:	Does this mean that drinking with your friend helps you not get depressed?
Charlie:	For sure.
Therapist:	I understand. What do you think are some negative consequences of drinking?
Charlie:	Well, it gets me into trouble sometimes (*laughs*).
Therapist:	Are you referring to the problems with your wife and boss?
Charlie:	Yes.
Therapist:	Can you tell me a bit more about these problems?
Charlie:	My wife threatens to leave me, and my boss wants to fire me if I don't do anything about it. That's why I am here, doc.
Therapist:	I understand. Tell me, how does it make you feel?
Charlie:	Frustrated. Angry.
Therapist:	I can imagine. So if I understand the situation correctly, it looks like drinking is a way for you to enjoy ties with your friends and perhaps also a way deal with loneliness and maybe depression in the short term. So drinking clearly has some positive short-term consequences. At the same time, drinking also has some potential longer-term negative personal, social, and professional consequences. Do I understand this correctly?

It can be very helpful to directly compare the positive and negative consequences of drinking and not drinking. Table 10.4 presents an example of some of these pros and cons. Listing the pros and cons of drinking and not drinking clarifies the factors that reinforce the drinking behaviors. It also provides an opportunity for the therapist to explore the short-term and long-term consequences of drinking. Of particular importance here are, obviously, the long-term negative consequences of drinking. The problems with his wife and his employer can easily lead to significant and undesirable consequences, such as, but not limited to, divorce, unemployment, poverty, and homelessness. Once Chuck realizes the negative consequences of his behavior, he may be ready to entertain the possibility of changing his behavior.

Table 10.4   The Pros and Cons of Drinking

	Pros	Cons
Drinking	Feeling good Part of friendship	Trouble with wife and boss Hangover
Not drinking	Better relationship with wife and boss Feeling better about myself	Not able to kick back with drink Not hanging out with buddies

Another motivational kernel is *choosing values*. Knowing the intrinsic qualities you are seeking in your life choices is more than merely goal setting (Chase et al., 2013). Even brief periods of writing about what is important to you in a given situation can motivate long-term change. Exploring sweet moments of life in detail, considering why you look up to your heroes, or examining what aspirations were violated in difficult life moments are all known to help clarify the personal values you want to adopt, which can serve as a powerful personal motivator.

SOME KERNELS TARGETING OVERT BEHAVIOR

The term "behavior" is a complicated construct that is differently defined based on the theoretical orientation. Modern behaviorists define this term very broadly to include all actions of a whole organism that can be thought of in terms of history and circumstance. Each of the psychological rows of the EEMM are, for them, types of action or "behavior" (e.g., emotional behavior; attentional actions). Most cognitively oriented therapists define "behavior" more narrowly to mean only overt behavior, as distinct from emotion, attention, and so on. Thus, when discussing behavioral phenomena, it is important to consider how the same words can land differently depending on the audience.

Psychological interventions targeting overt behaviors, such as *shaping* and *reinforcement*, are some of the most effective and reliable procedures. Systematically modifying maladaptive behaviors is always part of psychotherapy, and even a cursory review of these operant procedures would far exceed the limits of this chapter.

Behavioral activation is a powerful treatment kernel that is used to strengthen positive and more meaningful action patterns. People who experience low mood and anhedonia often become devoid of reinforcements, gratification, and pleasure. They may not have enough energy or voluntary attentional control to examine beliefs, automatic thoughts, and cognitive aspects that might maintain the depression. That may help explain why behavioral activation alone can have unexpectedly positive results, even with relatively severe affective problems. It is commonly recommended, especially at the beginning of treatment, in order to lift the patient's energy level and produce early treatment gains that can form a foundation for additional therapeutic work.

In the first step, the client is typically asked to monitor their activities during the week and record them on an activity log. In its simplest form, the activity log includes the time and date, location, a brief description of the activity, and a rating of how pleasant the activity was on a scale from 0 (not pleasant at all) to 100 (very pleasant). In the next step, the therapist and client often explore the reasons why some activities were pleasant and why others were rated as unpleasant. The goal is to build and increase the number of pleasant activities and to decrease the unpleasant activities and periods of inactivity during a normal week. In addition, it is desirable for the client to establish routines in their daily life and to implement regular eating and sleeping patterns.

Maladaptive behaviors are also often seen in the form of overt avoidance strategies focused on eliminating unpleasant states, subjective experiences, or biophysiological sensations. These strategies, however, maintain a maladaptive stance toward experiences and feed unhelpful emotional reasoning. Overt avoidance can be targeted through *exposure strategies* that produce organized contact with previously avoided events for the purposes of encouraging greater response flexibility.

SOME KERNELS TARGETING BIOPHYSIOLOGICAL PROCESSES

Diet, exercise, sex, and sleep are some of the biophysiological processes that are important contributors to psychological health. Many of the kernels discussed earlier also apply to these processes. Here, we focus on sleep as a case in point. *Sleep hygiene* refers to habits that affect one's quality of sleep, many of which we have discussed earlier. Below we provide sleep hygiene strategies that you can recommend to clients who have sleep problems (for more details, see Hofmann, 2011).

Improving Your Sleep Hygiene

1. Avoid drinking alcohol and caffeine (including soda and tea) and eating chocolate. If you can't avoid these altogether, don't consume them within four to six hours before you go to bed. Chocolate and caffeine are psychostimulants. Alcohol initially produces sleepiness; however, there is a stimulant effect a few hours later, when the blood alcohol level drops.

2. Avoid sugary, spicy, and heavy foods. If you can't avoid these altogether, don't eat those foods within four to six hours before you go to bed. Instead, eat light meals that are easy to digest (e.g., chicken, white rice, white bread, cooked vegetables, chicken soup, plain pasta).

3. Give yourself some time to unwind before bed and avoid doing strenuous mental activities right before bedtime.

4. Avoid dealing with emotionally arousing situations, including emotional movies, right before bedtime.

5. Make sure your bedroom is a pleasant environment. Your bed should feel comfortable. The bedroom should be a pleasant (cool) temperature, the right humidity, and well ventilated (i.e., should not be stuffy or smelly).

6. The bedroom should be dark and quiet. If there is a lot of distracting noise, try using earplugs or choose a different room.

7. Establish a sleeping ritual to implement before you go to bed. You may try any of the following: listen to a particular song or album (e.g., relaxing classical music or jazz), listen to the radio, or take a warm bath. Try not to watch TV because it can be too stimulating. Also, be careful with drinking liquid right before bedtime (such as a warm milk or tea) because this could interrupt your sleep later on if you need to get up in the middle of the night to go to the bathroom. If you find that drinking liquid immediately before bed does not disturb your sleep, try warm milk and honey.

8. Monitor which sleeping position works best for you. Some people find it easier to lie on their back; others prefer to lie on the right side. When lying on the left side, the heartbeat is more noticeable, which can be distracting to some people.

SOME KERNELS TARGETING THE SELF AND SOCIAL PROCESSES

Emotional and psychological health is associated with a positive bias to attribute positive events to oneself and negative events to other causes. This *self-serving attributional bias* seems to be missing or deficient in people with emotional problems, who tend to attribute negative events to internal (something about the self), stable (enduring), and global (general) causes (e.g., lack of ability, personality flaws). Such an attributional style implies that negative events are likely to recur in the future across a wide variety of domains, leading to widespread hopelessness. This breakdown of positive cognitive biases makes the world appear to be uncontrollable and unpredictable. Below is a story of Maria that illustrates these issues.

Maria's Mood

(adapted from Hofmann, 2011)

Maria is a thirty-nine-year-old woman who lives with her husband, Carlos, and thirteen-year-old son, Alex. She has a college degree in English literature and has not worked since Alex was born. Carlos works as an architect. Maria describes their marriage as sometimes "rocky." Although Carlos agrees that they occasionally have arguments, he does not think that they indicate any serious marital problems.

Maria has experienced depressive episodes since she was twenty-six years old, shortly after she gave birth to Alex. Since that time, her depression has reoccurred at least once each year, typically lasting six months or longer. Although often unpredictable, the episodes do tend to occur after major life changes, such as moving to a new home. During a depressive episode, she tends to withdraw from her family and experience strong feelings of emptiness and hopelessness. She perceives herself as being worthless, unlovable, and inadequate as a wife and blames herself for the problems in her marriage. She also loses interest in her hobbies (writing, reading, and going to theatrical plays with Carlos), loses her appetite, and spends a lot of time in bed, often wishing she could just disappear. During her depressive episodes, she feels unable to take care of basic responsibilities around the house. Maria and Carlos both feel that her depression often negatively affects their marriage and, conversely, that their disagreements—even minor ones—often trigger a depressive episode. The arguments reinforce her feelings of being worthless and unlovable, and she often believes that her husband is going to leave her, even though he has never threatened to. Maria has contemplated suicide as way to escape her feelings of emptiness, but she has never had a plan and says that she would never actually try to harm herself because she loves her family too much.

Although Maria loves her family and would do anything for her son, she felt that she had to give up a lot of her dreams by becoming a stay-at-home mom. During treatment, she remembered that her relationship with her father was very conflictual, and she often felt misunderstood and unloved by him. Although she does not think that her husband would ever leave her, she is worried that he will find another woman and abandon her. Maria realized that her fears of abandonment may have intruded into her relationship with her husband. Although the fights with her husband do not seem to be overly intense, she tends to ruminate about them excessively, even weeks after they have passed. Catastrophic beliefs (e.g., *My husband wants to leave me*) lead to withdrawal from social relationships and her marriage, exacerbating and perhaps even causing her depressive episode.

Stress is a common trigger for psychological distress, and interpersonal stressors can be especially powerful. Maria's strong negative self-concepts are evident (e.g., "I am worthless and unlovable"), but in her case, we might consider treatment kernels centering on *relationship-enhancement strategies* in which Maria and her husband can learn to express emotional needs more directly, to listen without withdrawal or criticism, to validate what is valid, and to create more secure attachments by relationship-enhancing activities.

THE FUTURE OF TREATMENT KERNELS

A large number of treatment kernels are readily available to clinicians to initiate treatment change by targeting therapeutic processes. We have only given a few examples here, and any list could not be exhaustive. Comprehensively organizing kernels into functional classes of intervention methods will require that the entire PBT research program (e.g., see Hofmann & Hayes, 2019) continue to progress. As a field we have had a good start, and we have discussed a wider variety of kernels elsewhere (Hayes & Hofmann, 2018), including those to target cognitive, affective, attentional, self-related, motivational, behavioral, biophysiological, and sociocultural processes.

As discussed in chapter 3, these processes are not independent. Instead, they are highly interactive, and any one kernel will often target a multitude of processes. Each kernel will need to be fitted to the client's specific needs, and some new kernels will need to be generated based on the client's particular problems, just as a builder might need to fabricate a window from scratch when design considerations demand it. Flexibility in PBT is key, for clients and therapists alike. PBT is a flexible process with two (or more) people being engaged in a dynamic interaction, similar to a playful dance with the therapist as the gently leading dancing partner. In the next chapter, we will illustrate this dance during PBT.

CHAPTER 11

The Course of Treatment

The course of treatment changes over time. In process-based therapy, we embrace the dynamic features of an individual's experience. For this matter, let's revisit the case of Maya. As you may remember, she was the client with chronic back pain due to a work accident. Our initial assessment revealed that she greatly focuses on her pain and worries that the pain will persist or that she might even reinjure herself, which could make the pain even worse. This has resulted in avoidance tendencies, restricting her occupational and social life. Maya felt that the accident and her pain was preventable, because it was caused by her employer, who was careless with implementing safety measures at her workplace. This left her being angry and resentful.

The therapist first thought that the most promising strategies to target her predominant symptoms—rumination and worrying, attention to pain and anger, and fear of reinjury—involved enhancing her level of mindfulness to detach from the unpleasant experience and targeting her negative repetitive cognitions. Therefore, the therapist taught Maya mindfulness skills so that she could learn to focus her attention in a more flexible and less judgmental way in order to stimulate healthy variation and flexible selection. The therapist's hope was that Maya would be able to direct her attention more deliberately rather than being controlled by her pain.

REVISITING THE NETWORK MODEL

Maya's therapist instructed her to mindfully observe her experience whenever her mind wanders toward her pain or other angry thoughts, images, feelings, or experiences. The therapist hoped that the factors that had previously been part of a maladaptive pattern would instead feed into an adaptive loop to strengthen her ability to direct her attention more adaptively. This is depicted again in figure 11.1. Introducing meditation practices was a critical therapeutic strategy to disturb Maya's maladaptive network. Her therapist hoped that this intervention would also enhance her sense of self-efficacy, shift her focus to valued goals rather than fear of reinjury, dampen her rumination, and lower her negative feelings toward the injury and her employer.

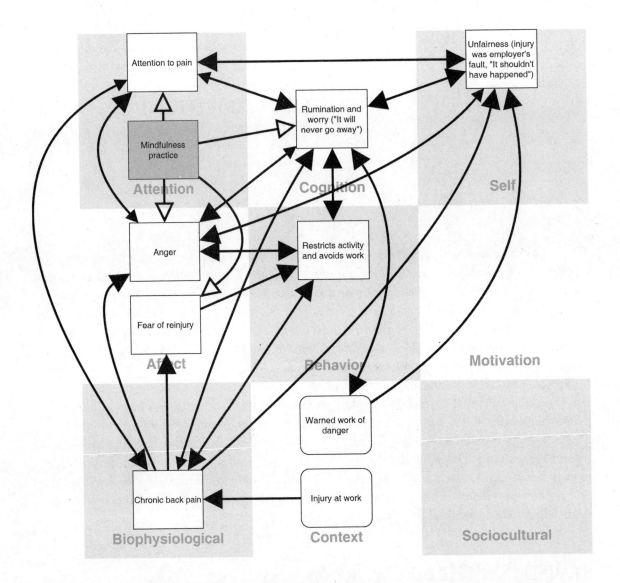

Figure 11.1 Hypothesized effect of mindfulness practice on Maya's network

Any therapy network is a dynamical system that changes with time. It is also a hypothetical set of assumptions that require empirical support. As such, a client's network is a temporary map that changes over the course of treatment and with the simple passage of time. Therefore, you will need to frequently check it to ensure not only that you and the client are both still on the right track but also whether the map needs to be redrawn. Once the initial network is determined you need to gather evidence to examine its validity.

GATHERING FEEDBACK TO GUIDE TREATMENT

The best way to gather accurate feedback is to collect high-density data of key measures that reflect the changes of the key nodes and their connections constituting the network. If the network reflects the hypothesis that a strong influence exists between two nodes, the measures assessing these nodes should then also show a strong relation. In Maya's case, the therapist assumed that the meditation practices would directly (and positively) affect her fear of injury, attention to pain, rumination and worry, and anger. In addition, the network reflects the therapist's hypothesis that the practices would enhance her focus on valued goals and her self-efficacy.

In order to gather some of this relevant data, the therapist first explored ways to measure some of these constructs. The most critical initial question in Maya's case is whether the mindfulness practices have the intended effect on fear of reinjury, rumination and worry, and anger.

Gathering such high-density data increases the burden for the client, which is why it can be useful to rely on technological tools. For example, a smartphone can collect a lot of potentially valuable data, especially when used in conjunction with biosensors (e.g., to measure heart rate variability or activity). Every smartphone already collects activity (such as steps during the day), gives geolocation, and keeps track of social contacts (such as the amount of engagement with certain social media apps or texting). The smartphone can also allow for active data gathering, for example by using an app that frequently asks the client to provide simple Likert-scale ratings of relevant network nodes (e.g., ratings of emotions on a 0–10 point scale). If you incorporate PBT into your clinical practice, we recommend that you integrate the potential of the smartphone into treatment as much as possible to collect high-density and valid data while minimizing client burden and maximizing client engagement. A low-tech version for gathering this information is of course a simple pen and paper monitoring of relevant information. For simplicity reasons, we chose this option here with Maya.

MAYA'S MEDITATION STRUGGLE

Therapist: Maya, as we discussed, there is a good possibility that mindfulness practices will lower your fear of reinjury, rumination and worry, and anger—or at least reduce their unwelcome impact. Are you still willing to try to establish a practice?

Maya: Sure. I'm interested. Let's try it.

Therapist: That's great. But why don't we make sure that the practices actually have the intended effect. This is a bit of a hassle because I will need to ask you to keep a record of some of these things.

Maya: Oh that's quite okay; I don't mind as long it's not too much work (*laughs*).

Therapist: It won't be. But it's quite important for us to understand how these things hang together. Once we understand it, we can effectively intervene. Makes sense?

Maya: Sure.

Therapist: Great. So let's keep it as straightforward as possible so we can minimize the time you spend on it while gathering the most important information to tailor your treatment. What do you think is most important to know based on the network we developed?

Maya: Definitely my pain. I want to feel less pain.

Therapist: Absolutely. So let's include a column of pain intensity. Let's say that you rate your pain intensity on a 0–10 point scale when you meditate. Let's take a look at the network. What else seems to be important that we should record to see if our network is accurate?

Maya: I guess that I am worried about reinjuring myself and that I am thinking about it a lot.

Therapist: I agree. So let's record the following about your mindfulness practice every day for the next two weeks (*hands client the form* [see table 11]).

Table 11.1   Portion of Maya's Monitoring Form

Day and Time	Duration of Meditation (min.)	Depth of Meditation (0–10)	Fear of Reinjury (0–10)	Rumination/Worry (0–10)	Anger (0–10)	Pain (0–10)
First: Second:						

Therapist: To determine whether mindfulness has the intended effect, I am asking you to meditate twice a day for the next two weeks and record how long you meditated, in minutes, and how deep the meditation was on a scale of 0 to 10, and then record your level of fear, rumination/worry, and anger during each practice. Please practice around the same time, once during the first half of the day and once sometime during the second half. Please schedule this at a time and place when you cannot be easily distracted by others. Do you have any questions?

Maya: No. I can do that. No problem.

Therapist: I realize that this is a lot to do, but for the next two weeks, we really need to do this in order to determine if we are on the right track. Otherwise, we are wasting our time at best, or we might make things even worse. So it's very important that we gather this data. Do you anticipate any problems?

Maya: No. No problem.

Therapist: Great. Thank you. Do you already know when and where you can find time to do this?

DISCUSSING THE FEEDBACK

Regardless of the data type and source, the collected data needs to be carefully examined in the next step. Traditional CBT routinely involves gathering similar data, yet on a much less frequent basis. This data is then often used as a brief check of whether treatment has an effect on the client's presenting problem.

In PBT, this data has a much more important function. It is used to examine the functionality of different problems, for example, by examining the covariation pattern of the ratings. In the simplest case, this is done by examining whether changes in one variable are consistently associated with changes in the other variable in the expected direction. The overall trend (e.g., improvement over time) is considerably less important than the covariation pattern between the measures that are assumed to form a causal relationship.

As part of the intervention, the therapist and Maya decided to try meditation in order to disturb her maladaptive network. The hypothesis was that introducing regular meditation practices would enhance her level of mindfulness and reduce her fear of reinjury, rumination and worry, and anger associated with her injury. Maya's monitoring, however, revealed a very different pattern (see table 11.2.).

Table 11.2   Maya's Completed Monitoring Form—Week 1

Day and Time	Duration of Meditation (min.)	Depth of Meditation (0–10)	Fear of Reinjury (0–10)	Rumination/Worry (0–10)	Anger (0–10)	Pain (0–10)
First: Wed, 9 a.m.	10	5	9	9	9	9
Second: Wed, 3 p.m.	10	5	9	8	9	9
First: Thurs, 9 a.m.	15	6	9	9	9	9
Second: Thurs, 4 p.m.	15	6	8	9	9	9
First: Fri, 9 a.m.	20	6	8	9	9	9
Second: Fri, 3 p.m.	20	6	9	9	9	9
First: Sat, 10 a.m.	30	7	8	9	9	9
Second: Sat, 2 p.m.	30	7	8	9	9	9
First: Sun, 10 a.m.	30	7	9	9	9	9
Second: Sun, 2 p.m.	30	6	9	9	9	9
First: Mon, 9 a.m.	10	5	9	9	9	9
Second: Mon, 4 p.m.	10	6	9	9	9	9
First: Tues, 8 a.m.	20	6	9	9	9	9
Second: Tues, 6 p.m.	20	6	8	9	8	9

Although Maya practiced mediation regularly, her fear of reinjury, rumination/worry, and anger remained virtually unchanged. Her therapist and she discussed this in the next session to examine the effect of meditation on her emotional state.

Therapist: Thank you for doing the meditation practices and filling out the form. How was that?

Maya: Thanks. Well, I think it went okay. I had trouble sitting for so long in a stretch, but eventually I got the hang of it.

Therapist: Great. How did you like the meditation practices?

Maya: I don't know. I am sorry to say, but I don't think it works. It really didn't do much for my pain and my concerns around it. But maybe it just needs much more time and maybe I should just keep trying.

Therapist: That's certainly a possibility. Maybe we should just keep trying it for a little longer and see how it goes. But it's also possible that this is simply not the right approach for you, and we want to make sure that we are choosing the right strategy for your problem. What do you think? Should we take a close look at it first before we decide to keep going?

Maya: Sure, makes sense.

It is possible that through repeated mindfulness practice, Maya might learn to respond to her pain differently and to redirect her attentional focus to adaptive stimuli. However, it is unclear if and when this beneficial effect of mindfulness can be expected. Without clear and immediate benefits, pursuing this practice for Maya can lead to worsening of her problems, discourage and frustrate her and the therapist, and even heighten the risk of her discontinuing treatment prematurely. Instead of pushing forward with a usually beneficial but in Maya's case questionable strategy, the PBT therapist reexamines the approach.

PROBING THE NETWORK

If a network reflects the hypothesis that two nodes are strongly connected, then changes in the measure of one node should be consistently associated with changes in the measure of the other node. If they are associated, we can retain the network for the time being (until it changes again). If this is not the case, then the nodes are measured inaccurately and/or the nodes are not directly connected.

Remember that mere association does not imply causation. However, our network makes assumptions about the directionality and therefore also about the causality of the association. Exploring the cause-effect relationship between nodes often requires some detailed discussions in therapy sessions. Sometimes, the effect is more obvious than at other times. For example, it is quite evident that Maya's fear of reinjury is caused by her chronic back pain and that her back pain causes her to ruminate and worry. Many other nodes in Maya's network are bidirectional, but the causality of the two nodes is sometimes asymmetrical (e.g., rumination causes Maya to feel angry, and anger also causes her to ruminate but to lesser degree). When using smartphone data or biosensor data, we can examine the temporal relationship between two measures in order to determine the directionality and causality of measures.

Demonstrating causality can be difficult if there is a significant time-lagged influence of one variable on another variable. For example, sleep problems the night before might cause low mood the next day even though the client is not aware of this association, in part because of the time delay. Monitoring relevant data, examining the covariation pattern, and determining directionality and causality can bring great clarity to a problem and provide an opportunity to effectively intervene.

Therapist: I want to better understand why meditating is not helping and may even make things worse. This can clarify the process we need to focus on. Could we please do the meditation here in session and you share with me every thought and image that pops into your mind as you do it? It might be easiest if I could ask you at various points what you are thinking this very moment. So when I ask, "Now?" I want you to verbalize and tell me your thoughts, images, or experiences you have at this very moment as you are doing the practice. You don't need to give an elaborate answer. You could just say something like "focus on breath" or "hear sound" or "tingling in leg," etcetera. I will ask you "Now?" at pretty random intervals every few minutes. Makes sense?

Maya: Yes.

Therapist: Great. Go!

Maya: (*Meditates*)

Therapist: (*after about two minutes*) Now?

Maya: Breath more slowly.

Therapist: Great. (*after about two minutes*) Now?

Maya: Breath more slowly.

Therapist: Okay (*takes notes...after about two minutes*) Now?

Maya: Back hurts.

Therapist: Okay *(takes notes…after about two minutes)* Now?

Maya: Frustrated that back hurts. I need to shift position to make it less painful.

Maya responded to the therapist's prompts with thoughts and images relating to the present moment, but she also continuously endorsed a focus on pain-related statements, such as "Back hurts," or "I need to shift position to make it less painful."

It became clear that the mindfulness practice focused her attention on her pain. Therefore, the mindfulness practice did not have the intended and hypothesized influence on Maya's problems related to fear of reinjury, rumination/worry, and anger. In contrast, it inadvertently seemed to exacerbate the problem. It might be possible to work more on how to meditate to avoid these problems, but a change in direction could yield more immediate benefits.

This example highlights an important feature of PBT: utilizing the therapy session as an experimental arena rather than as a traditional consulting session that is more detached from the client's actual experience. The approach of PBT is to try it out here and now and bring the therapist into the entire process.

REDRAWING THE NETWORK ON THE FLY

Trying out meditation and monitoring its effects on her fear, rumination/worry, and anger was a valuable experience despite its showing that it was not the right strategy for Maya at the present time. Bringing the practice into the session showed that the meditation practice raised her attention on the pain experience.

PBT follows the EEMM principle of variation, selection, and retention in a given context on all levels. Here, the therapist *varied* different strategies that were guided by evidence and sound theoretical models (i.e., mindfulness practice decreases fear and anger by reducing rumination and worry). However, because the meditation strategy did not have the intended effect, the therapist chose not to *select* it and *retain* the strategy by asking Maya to continue with the practice. Instead of considering it a failure, they used the experience to further understand the nature of Maya's problem.

The therapist redrew Maya's network with her help to include the actual role of the meditation practice (see figure 11.2). As reflected in the network, meditation had the unintended effect of enhancing her fear of injury, rumination and worry, anger, and even back pain itself. It is possible that meditation is directly related to these experiences or indirectly linked through enhancing her attention to the pain experience. Bringing it into the therapy session provides some support for the latter.

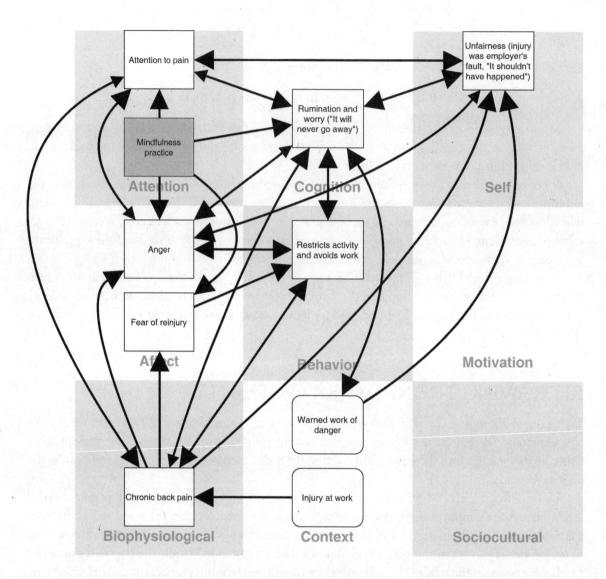

Figure 11.2 When Maya's mindfulness practice does not have the intended effect

SELECTING A NEW STRATEGY

Of course, it is quite possible that the initial strategy (mindfulness practice) would have a very different effect with a different client or with more effort. If meditation had shown signs of more effectiveness, the therapist would have worked with Maya to find ways to maximize its benefits and to retain the practice (e.g., by establishing a practice regimen). However, therapists should be prepared to show a maximum degree of flexibility in choosing the strategy that is most adaptive for a given client in the given context. In Maya's case, it didn't work as intended. This is not to say that the therapist "goes back to the drawing board" each time a strategy hits a bump in the road. The prior strategy was not a "failure"—it was a step forward in understanding the nature of the client's problem. This is illustrated in the dialogue below.

Therapist: Does this network and its influence of mindfulness make sense?

Maya: Yes, I am afraid it does.

Therapist: I really don't think you need to be sorry about it. We learned something very important: meditation raises your pain and anger, and even your fear of reinjury, rumination/worry, and attention to pain. What do you think the process is through which this happens? How come meditating raises your pain experience?

Maya: Well, maybe I am not doing it right.

Therapist: I think you are doing great. Really. We were able to show that this practice, which can be quite helpful, is not working for you in your current situation. Maybe later it will work for you. But not now. So why do you think we are getting the effect we are getting?

Maya: It seems like I am concentrating too much on my pain. It's always with me. It's constantly there. I can't escape. Just sitting there makes it worse because my mind just goes there.

Therapist: It makes a lot of sense. So we could even redraw the network to show that meditation raises your attention toward pain, which in turn raises your pain experience, anger, etcetera. Is that right?

Maya: Yes.

Therapist: Okay. Knowing that, what could help you with your pain?

Maya: Well, if my mind is not constantly focused on it.

Therapist: I agree. It's very difficult to not think of something when you don't want to think of it. For example, if I told you not to think of a white bear, this white bear would turn into an intrusive image *(therapist illustrates it)*. What we can do, however, is to take some vacation from your worrying. What do you think?

Maya: That would be great! But how I would I do that?

A number of possible options are feasible here. Some of the most effective core treatment strategies or core therapeutic competencies (which, you'll recall, we call *treatment kernels*) have been described in detail in our book *Process-Based CBT* (see Hayes & Hofmann, 2018), in which we designated a chapter to each kernel with concrete practical tips.

There is no absolute right or wrong answer. But some of these kernels will be more beneficial than others. In fact, many kernels will not be suitable in Maya's case because they do not target the underlying process and will therefore not disturb her network. Often, more than one kernel might be suitable, and often a suitable kernel targets more than one process and more than one node in the network. Below is a list of common, evidence-based treatment kernels.

Treatment Kernels

Contingency management	Cognitive reappraisal
Stimulus control	Modifying core beliefs
Shaping	Cognitive defusion
Self-management	Experiential acceptance
Problem solving	Attentional training
Arousal reduction	Values choice and clarification
Coping/Emotion regulation	Mindfulness practice
Exposure	Enhancing motivation
Behavioral activation	Crisis management
Interpersonal skills	

These kernels are organized into fairly large units, and we would hope that all therapists, regardless of their orientation, would be familiar with all of them. PBT encourages you to choose the most suitable kernel to most effectively move the underling process in a particular client in a given context, and that is not possible if only a very limited set can be deployed. Before even talking to a client, a more traditionally oriented behavior therapist might be more inclined to focus on exposure, stimulus control, and shaping; an ACT therapist on values work and defusion; a traditional CBT therapist on cognitive reappraisal; and so on. That does not make sense. All of these methods can fit within most evidence-based therapy models. What needs to drive kernel use is client need based on a process-based functional analysis.

Action Step 11.1   Choosing a Treatment Kernel

Let's take another look at the problem you have chosen for yourself and examine which treatment kernels are most appropriate for you. Please indicate the target(s) for each intervention and indicate the likelihood of success on a 0–10 point scale.

Treatment Kernel	Target(s)	Likelihood of Success (0–10)
Contingency management		
Stimulus control		
Shaping		
Self-management		
Problem solving		
Arousal reduction		
Coping/Emotion regulation		
Exposure		
Behavioral activation		

Treatment Kernel	Target(s)	Likelihood of Success (0–10)
Interpersonal skills		
Cognitive reappraisal		
Modifying core beliefs		
Cognitive defusion		
Experiential acceptance		
Attentional training		
Values choice and clarification		
Mindfulness practice		
Enhancing motivation		
Crisis management		

Example

To illustrate how to use this table as a guide to select treatment kernels, consider our client with social anxiety whose completed table looked like the one below. It would make perfect sense to focus on the kernels rated 8 and 9 over those with 5s.

Treatment Kernel	Target(s)	Likelihood of Success (0–10)
Exposure	Exposure to social situations that provoke fear and nervousness.	7
Modifying core beliefs	Modify the belief that there are "winners and losers," that "I'm a loser," that "I have to proof myself."	8
Cognitive defusion	Defuse from painful thoughts that "I'm a loser."	7
Experiential acceptance	Practice acceptance of feelings of fear and nervousness.	9
Attentional training	Practice flexibly adjusting my focus outward to other people.	5
Values choice and clarification	Clarify what matters to me, as a focus point in social situations.	5
Mindfulness practice	Practice being present with myself, my emotions, in the here and now.	8

Returning to Maya's case, we have already chosen meditation as a mindfulness practice in order to target reduction of—or at least better contextual control over—her fear of reinjury, rumination and worry, anger, and pain experience. Attentional processes still seem important, but the treatment kernel we initially chose moved it in the wrong direction. What the therapist did was to target attention in another way, as we'll see in this next conversation segment.

Therapist: Let's designate a time when you worry about your pain. Let's say maybe two hours from 2 to 4 p.m. every day. You can worry as much as you want during these two hours, but you have a worry vacation outside of this worry time. So if you have an urge to worry about your pain in the morning, put it off until 2 p.m., when you can worry as much as you want for two hours. What do you say?

Maya: Interesting. I don't think I want to worry for two full hours. But let's try it.

Therapist: Before we do that, however, let's see what we hope would happen to the network if you have a worry vacation. Do you agree with this network? *(hands client the figure below* [figure 11.3].

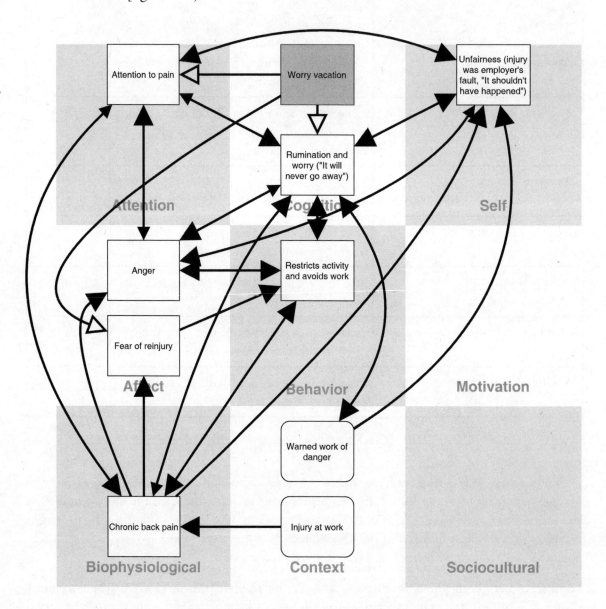

Figure 11.3 Effect of Maya's worry vacation

Worry vacation (a positive reformulation of worry time intervention) was not a specific kernel on the list of treatment kernels shown above. It is a strategy that includes primarily kernels of attentional training and to some extent stimulus control and self-management. These kernels are the basic building blocks for the specific treatment strategies targeting the specific process in Maya's case. Even though this option is not a frequently used kernel, the impact on the targeted process should be rapid and evident—so we have not left an empirically focused approach.

GATHERING MORE FEEDBACK

Together with Maya, the therapist examined whether the proposed process is, in fact, valid—namely whether "worry vacation" is associated with less rumination and worry, attention to pain, and fear of reinjury. If so, this should then reduce her anger and intensity of the pain experience (indirectly, but perhaps even directly). Another two-week high-density monitoring phase would clarify these assumptions and might require another network modification if necessary.

Therapist: What should we measure to see if this new network is accurate?

Maya: We could see if the worry vacation is helpful.

Therapist: Great idea. Let's record the following every day for the next two weeks (*hands client the form below* [table 11.3]). First, I want you to use this monitoring sheet to record your worry-free time; how good you are feeling, from 0, not good at all, to 10, very good; your fear of reinjury on a scale of 0, which means no fear, to 10, which means extreme fear; how much you ruminate and worry, from 0 to 10; and your level of anger, from 0 to 10.

Table 11.3   Portion of Maya's Monitoring Form

Day and Time	Worry Vacation (min.)	Feeling Good (0–10)	Fear of Reinjury (0–10)	Rumination/Worry (0–10)	Anger (0–10)	Pain (0–10)
First: Second:						

The purpose of this monitoring form is to examine whether the intervention has the intended effect. In other words, will having a worry vacation be associated with better mood, less fear of reinjury, and also less worrying, anger, and pain? If it indeed has the intended effect, Maya should retain this simple strategy and even further build on it. If it is not successful after giving it a good chance to work, other strategies should be considered. Eventually, PBT moves from simple to more complex processes. Here is how.

MOVING TOWARD MORE COMPLEX PROCESSES

The intervention we just selected could be beneficial by providing Maya with short-term relief from her pain through targeting repetitive negative thinking, including worry and rumination. These are specific cognitive processes related to her pain experience.

Once Maya feels that she is able to manage her pain and has greater control over these cognitive processes related to pain, other intervention strategies that target more complex processes may be considered. These might include those targeting the self and social issues by participating in the worker's union and engaging in other behaviors that move her toward her valued goals, as we already discussed. Other important strategies that the therapist should consider for Maya are those aimed at rebuilding her social network and her quality of life, which have been impaired by her pain. This may include doing regular morning exercises with her neighbor and engaging in other social activities. As they did for the meditation practice, the therapist and Maya should carefully evaluate and test the impact of each strategy in order to identify and measure the proposed process through which the intervention might work.

If an intervention does not have the intended effect and does not target the right process for a client, you will need to flexibly explore other treatment kernels to find the most suitable approach to a given client in the given context. As much as possible, these strategies should not be restricted to homework assignments; the processes should also be played out in your office. We discourage roleplays and instead encourage you to be mindful and catch a process in the session whenever it happens.

You can use the guiding questions below to help you determine the best treatment kernels for a particular client in a particular context and make the necessary shifts along the way based on the feedback you and your client gather.

Guiding Questions – Course of Treatment

Understand the Problem

- What are the main problems/critical nodes?

- How are the nodes functionally connected?

- Where are the self-sustaining and positive feedback loops?

- Have all EEMM dimensions been considered?

Plan the Treatment

- What are the short-term goals?

- What are the long-term goals?

- What are the elements in the network that prohibit or interfere with these goals?

- What are possible strategies to intervene effectively?

Implement Strategies

- How do you tailor a particular strategy to the client's particular network?

- How do you ensure that the strategy is implemented correctly?

- Can the strategy be practiced in your office?

- How do you monitor the implementation?

Examine Effect of Strategy on Network

- How do you best quantify the change?

- Is the change process moving along in the expected direction?

- Do the nodes show the expected degree of covariation (and directionality)?

- Should the strategy/network be revisited/revised?

CHAPTER 12

From Problems to Prosperity: Maintaining and Expanding Gains

Evidence-based therapies have long focused on the importance of "programming for maintenance" in clinical work. Classic examples include anticipating and planning for slips; adding exposure to situations, emotions, or thoughts that likely could lead to resurgence of past problems; and adding incentives or supports to help sustain motivation (e.g., public commitment strategies, public posting of progress). Entire intervention approaches, such as "relapse prevention," have emerged to address maintenance issues.

These classic approaches to maintenance are step one, but more can be said based on a process-based approach. Maintenance in a PBT approach requires a shift in focus for both the client and the therapist. Maintenance successes from a PBT point of view involve

1. focusing on processes over immediate outcomes;

2. building self-sustaining loops that support healthy processes of change;

3. practicing and repeating key processes of change;

4. integrating these healthy processes into larger patterns of action; and

5. establishing reemergence of problem areas as cues for positive processes of change.

In this chapter we will explore each of these five aspects of a successful maintenance approach.

FOCUSING ON PROCESSES OVER IMMEDIATE OUTCOMES

The proximal "outcomes" in a PBT approach are processes themselves. It matters *how* change happens, not just *that* change happens, because in the future positive process skills will allow the person to evolve their lives on purpose.

Suppose two students are studying for an exam, and both end up getting the same high score. The first student did not know the topic very well at first but studied hard with a peer and challenged herself with test questions and practice exams until she was confident that she knew the material. The second student had a "knack" for the topic, and his sister had taken the same class two years earlier and predicted accurately what would likely be on the exam.

Which of these two students would you predict would get a good grade in the next class? If you predict based on outcomes alone, both would be equally likely, but any thoughtful person will predict that the first student would be better positioned for future success because the source of the good grade is more reliable and in the person's control. So it is with processes of change.

That same point helps explain why people often develop recalcitrant problems to begin with. All human beings develop skills over time, and it would be logical to believe that they all get better and better at accomplishing their goals over time by trial and error. That would be logical, but it would be wrong because people can learn the wrong lesson from experience alone. Generally unhelpful processes of change often produce positive outcomes over the short and even medium term. This can strengthen those largely negative processes, and the person will use them at other times and in other places, to their long-term detriment. The means matter as much as the outcome.

For example, suppose a person feels a deep sense of inadequacy. He may fear he is unwanted, unable, and unlovable. To escape this painful state, he drives himself to achieve, using internal threats and demands, while hiding these deeper emotions and beliefs, certain that no one would want to be around him if such vulnerabilities were evident. Yes, "success" may follow—even a whipped horse may reach a destination—but this "success" will ring hollow because instead of being able to enjoy his growing competence, he will spiral one step deeper into a growing sense of inadequacy and aloneness despite his competence. Worse in a way, "success" will cement the processes in place, and then, at other times and places in which healthier process skills are needed, such as when building genuine relationships, he will fall back on processes that cannot produce the desired outcome.

Clients and therapists can both easily be fooled by outcomes alone, and there is a human tendency to grasp at immediate outcomes even if it is not wise in the long run. This is made worse when deliberately creating psychological change because, in the world of outcomes, sometimes things superficially need to get worse before they get better. Metaphorically, if a glass has a thick settled layer of dirt in the bottom, cleaning it will stir things up, and for a few moments the glass will appear to be worse than ever. If a couple needs to have hard conversations about difficult material that spans several years, you can expect that sometimes the conversations will be heated, conflictual, or painful, even if the process itself is broadly healthy. Any evidence-based therapist knows of such examples: extinction bursts, the short relapse often seen in the early stages of cognitive therapy for depression that marks a deeper engagement, difficult emotions during exposure, and so on. In situations like these, if the client and therapist maintain processes themselves as proximal outcomes, over and above short-term outcomes per se, the client is better set up to take steps that feed into an overall pattern of progress.

Consider a person with social anxiety who is about to give a speech. Healthy steps such as practicing beforehand, maintaining a greater degree of mindful awareness, and emotional openness will help the person focus on what works and what doesn't, increasing the likelihood of speaking success over the long term. "Above all, just focus on being present," a process-oriented therapist might say, helping processes themselves become the primary outcome focus. An unwise therapist might focus more on the features of the speech itself, even if that connotes the unhealthy suggestion that the speaker can and should eliminate anxiety.

It is worth noting here that a process-focused approach to creating robust and lasting change can be applied to the therapist themself. One of the major strengths of a process-based approach is that focusing on processes of change helps give immediate feedback to the practitioner. The more common focus is the therapeutic alliance and positive symptom change as reported by clients. But both of these are weaker guides than properly selected processes of change, either because they are more delayed or because they are less precise.

The therapeutic alliance typically relates to outcomes, but it does so primarily because good alliances model and instigate positive processes of change, such as having greater self-compassion, being less self-judgmental, or taking a more active stance toward one's life situation. We know that is true because when healthy change processes are allowed to compete statistically with the therapeutic alliance, the alliance is commonly no longer a significant mediator of change (e.g., Gifford et al., 2011). Said in another way, the alliance is a means to an end, and the "end" is the internalization of healthy processes of change that are modeled and supported in the therapeutic relationship.

Symptom change alone as a proximal outcome is worrisome because it can occur through suppression or through other means that do not predict future success. Thus, taking a "process is the proximal outcome" focus can help not just the client but also the therapist because it gives therapists the best and most reliable proximal information, according to intervention science, about how therapy is progressing. This is why we have called for the development of short session-by-session process measures that can be applied longitudinally—and fortunately these are now appearing (e.g., Probsta et al., 2020).

Broadly focused and long-term outcomes are a different matter, as a metric for both the therapist and the clients. If they are in accord with the client's true goals, broadly focused and long-term outcomes are indeed the final arbiter of effectiveness. Do not mindlessly confuse such outcomes with long-term level of signs or symptoms, however. The traditional psychiatric nosology is far too narrowly focused and has no right to override client choices about their purposes, so unless a client chooses reduction of those symptoms as their broad and long-term goal, signs and symptoms should not be assumed to be of central relevance to the ultimate outcomes being sought. Carefully chosen outcomes based on client choice are the ultimate arbiter of treatment, but usually, by definition, they are a poor proximal guide to clinicians, and thus they are only likely to be of relevance in organized research.

BUILDING SELF-SUSTAINING LOOPS THAT SUPPORT HEALTHY PROCESSES OF CHANGE

Evolving is purposely fostered by aligning contextually apt variation and selective retention with the right process of change. Self-sustaining loops are the clear sign of that alignment. For example, if the person who is anxious about making a speech focuses on "being present" during a talk, they may notice when their attention wanders or when entangling thoughts arise. If process skills are available to redirect their attention or to allow challenging thoughts to pass by in favor of more helpful thoughts, not only is the likelihood of a successful speech increased, so too is the likelihood of deploying such process skills next time in other talks or in other communicative situations. A self-amplifying set of relationships can then be strengthened in which seeking out opportunities to speak, practicing and preparing, staying present, deploying healthy psychological processes, and pursuing better jobs gradually leads to competence and confidence in such situations.

Network thinking is helpful in this aspect of treatment planning. The therapist needs to think about what the possible naturally sustaining consequences of positive process changes would be. If they exist in the client's life, how can these healthy process changes be tied to them? If they do not exist, how can they be created?

For example, suppose a client with a trauma history is learning to take in the perspective of others and to use this skill to deepen his mindful awareness of his own needs as well. Practicing compassionate listening can support self-compassion if that link is built deliberately, but if the person is socially isolated, there is no place for this to occur. On the other hand, seeking out an advocacy role with abused children might allow the client to create a self-sustaining loop in which showing more kindness and awareness to himself supports and serves as a model for that work with children, and being compassionate toward the children might support and sustain patterns of self-compassion. Self-sustaining helpful loops can be identified or sought out in much the same way that self-sustaining unhelpful loops are identified in process-based functional analysis.

PRACTICING AND REPEATING KEY PROCESSES OF CHANGE

The single most important retention process for psychological processes of change is repetition. "Having a practice" is a common phrase among people who meditate, but there is no reason it should not be a mantra for those trying to learn all healthy processes of change, from reappraisal skills to values, from self-efficacy to self-acceptance. Meta-analyses long ago showed that homework and deliberate practice foster positive outcomes of evidence-based therapy. Building process-focused homework and deliberate practice into intervention is a key feature of PBT for that reason. You will note that throughout this volume we have asked you, as a reader, to practice new skills and have done so in an incremental series of action steps that build upon one another. The same should apply to your clients.

INTEGRATING THESE HEALTHY PROCESSES INTO LARGER PATTERNS OF ACTION

Action patterns have their own momentum—the best predictor of future action is past action because psychological adjustments occur repeatedly. Acquiring a new skill may require special focus, but retaining a skill involves learning how to deploy it when needed, even when it is *not* in focus. A good way to do that is to link new ways of doing things to existing positive habits. For example, suppose a process-based therapist is teaching a client to do a quick one-minute-long body scan at the start of the day to detect any emotional issues that are being needlessly carried over from the previous day. If that client always gets a cup of coffee in the morning and reads the paper, it might be best to try to link the body scan to the moment the coffee cup hits the table and the client sits in their chair. This can be done by practice until it is integrated into one larger pattern.

Usually, clients will have a mental list of things they do almost every day—things that are simply not "optional." These are great "planter box" areas to use to grow new process seeds.

ESTABLISHING REEMERGENCE OF PROBLEM AREAS AS CUES FOR POSITIVE PROCESSES OF CHANGE

Psychological change is not smooth—it's up and down. Rather than wait for "relapse," it is best to consider where and how a stable system might break down and where it would likely be seen. One of the more reliable indications of a change in a dynamical system is "flicker"—brief periods in which relationships within a network shift and then return to a previous state.

You have probably noticed this phenomenon when trying to establish a habit. For example, if you have a new diet in which, say, you swear to yourself you will avoid sugar and high carbohydrate foods, you may catch yourself unexpectedly grabbing a small sweet as you pass through the kitchen, just hours or days before crashing out of the diet altogether.

Dynamical systems analysis has shown that flicker can predict large-scale system change both in a positive and negative direction. Clinicians are intuitively aware of this. A practitioner working on greater emotional openness will catch a watery eye or quivering lip and know that an opportunity for growth is available. A practitioner doing parent training will teach a parent how to "catch their child being good" so that small steps in the right direction can be noticed and built upon.

Clinicians should be on the lookout for positive and negative flicker in session, but clients too can learn to notice these same signs. Tiny slips or risky, apparently irrelevant actions can be integrated into a vigorous reemphasis of processes of change when they are detected. For example, a careful look at the single instance of grabbing a treat from a counter may reveal a thought like *I deserve a treat since I've been so good with my eating for so long and I finally have made real gains.* This cognitive pattern ("I get to break the rules because I'm owed") may be itself quite old and entrenched. It could have a long history of almost childlike self-indulgence.

With a small tweak, a wise therapist could help establish a similar but more helpful cognitive pattern (e.g., "I should be good to myself when I've made hard changes" and "I should be good to myself when I stick to my word—but not by violating it"). That kind of awareness could foster a healthier pattern of noticing the pull to slip and using a deliberate "treat" to support a desired pattern, such as buying a small piece of clothing or scheduling a visit to the spa when the "I'm owed" thoughts show up.

APPLYING RULES OF MAINTENANCE

It is worth reminding you how these five features were applied earlier in this book. Take the case of Maya, the client with chronic pain who had been injured at work and was entangled in rumination, anger, a sense of unfairness, and restriction of activity. Mindfulness and, in the "do-over," a worry vacation were deployed to inhibit or regulate rumination, fear of reinjury, and attention to pain, largely through these two different ways of targeting attentional processes. It's worth noticing, however, that while attentional processes targeting these aspects were key, other parts of her network would likely be untouched by attentional flexibility alone, especially restriction of activity and a sense of unfairness. The therapist used a focus on valued goals to help generate a habit of exercising with her neighbor and involvement with a worker's union to help give meaning and a behavior target to Maya's experiences and the sense of unfairness they contained. Maya's therapist focused on emotional openness and a greater sense of her health needs to encourage the exercise—that's an example of a *focus on processes of change* over immediate exercise outcomes per se.

The linkage to the daily exercise with a neighbor has the possibility of *repetition*, linked to a positive socially rewarding experience. That will not just help put purpose back into her life, but will help put more life into her healthy purposes—building a kind of *self-sustaining feedback loop*. Her new ways of responding to thoughts and feelings can enter into this exercise and social pattern, building a larger or more *integrative action pattern* that will be more resistant to change. The therapist even *anticipated that anger might emerge* to disrupt the pattern but encouraged the client to see that anger is also a useful cue since it can hide positive motivation. Thus, all five of the features we have described were included in that plan.

LIFE IS A PROCESS TO BE LIVED, NOT A PROBLEM TO BE SOLVED

One of the profound lessons of process-based therapy is that therapy is not a "one and done." Therapy is not just for the one out of five people carrying a standard psychiatric diagnosis. Instead, processes of change can become guides to human growth and resilience. In other words, processes of change can become a "five out of five" toolkit of life enhancement and empowerment methods, organized under a "problems to prosperity" vision.

No one would think to tell a person with a physical health problem, "Oh dear! I guess now you need to exercise!" Yet, oddly, that is exactly what is most common in the area of mental health and resilience. There is a simple reason: the latent disease model misleads the public and practitioners alike. A process-based approach invites another way forward because, in area after area, research is showing that healthy processes of change that are being identified in intervention science can be deployed to foster positive life changes as well. By recognizing the broader implications of adaptive process-based changes, we are better able to "broaden and build" these adaptive processes.

Applied psychology has long known that people who are resilient, growing, flexible, and socially connected are less likely to fall into mental health problems and are more likely to rise to important life challenges. That effect exists in part because healthy processes of change are responsible for positive growth.

In PBT we can use the EEMM to help apply processes of change to positive life growth, not just mental health problems. Even if the original reason for consultation was purely "problem oriented," before concluding work with a client, you should consider each of the top six rows of the EEMM in terms of psychologically positive processes of change and the aspirational goals of the client. You should then do the same for the sociocultural level of the EEMM, examining especially the person's friendships, family, and intimate relationships. Finally, you should consider the biophysiological level of the EEMM.

In each row of the EEMM, look for healthy variation, selection, and retention in context and consider what could best move your client toward the greater prosperity they yearn for, using process skills learned in therapy to look at growth from a "broaden and build" perspective. In some systems of care, this kind of work cannot continue for very long because the health care system is not actually health oriented but rather is just focused on treating illnesses, and payment for work of this kind is restricted.

For that reason, in current systems of care, often this work has to go on under the rubric of relapse prevention, discharge planning, programming maintenance and generalization, and the like. In other systems, work on mental and behavioral health prevention, work effectiveness, leadership, teamwork, diversity training, weight loss, smoking cessation, injury prevention, and so on can provide ways to build in resources for implementing the "problems to prosperity" vision that is implicit in PBT.

By now you are highly familiar with the psychological rows of the EEMM, so we need not re-present those here, but we have had less to say about how sociocultural and biophysiological processes might be addressed. In table 12.1 we show a version of a sociocultural EEMM, focused on dyads and intimate relationships, which lends itself to this phase of process-based work almost regardless of the original presenting problem. For sake of illustration, the model we will exemplify to give life to this idea of using socially extended psychological processes to focus on prosperity goals is drawn from the psychological flexibility model that is used in ACT.

Table 12.1   Socially Extended Adaptive Psychological Flexibility Processes

Copyright Steven C. Hayes. Used by permission.

		Healthy Variation	Selection Criteria	Retention	Context
Group Dimensions	Cognitive	Mutual understanding	Functional coherence	Broaden and build using practice, and integration into larger patterns	Use conscious attention to maintain balance
	Affective	Compassion	Feeling		
	Self	Attachment and conscious connection	Belonging		Key strength of this process
	Attentional	Joint attention	Orientation		
	Motivational	Shared values and acknowledgment	Meaning	Key strength of these processes	Use monitoring to detect maintenance of values-based commitment
	Overt Behavior	Shared commitments	Competence		

What this dyadic EEMM shows is that it is not hard to enhance flexibility skills in the cognitive, affective, self, attentional, motivational, and overt behavioral dimensions and to socially extend them. In a psychological flexibility model, the flexibility skills of defusion, acceptance, a perspective-taking sense of self, flexible attention to the now, values, and committed action can be readily extended to social processes of change in the areas of mutual understanding, compassion, attachment and conscious connection, joint attention, shared values and acknowledgment, and shared commitments. This provides a kind of roadmap for how to move from a problem focus to a prosperity focus, using processes of change as a guide.

Suppose a client has been helped in a PBT approach by establishing great acceptance and defusion skills, linked to a program of values-based exposure. On the other side of that work, the client has a new set of process-based skills. As such, the client can more readily share values with others and deploy acceptance and defusion skills to help build greater degrees of social compassion and mutual understanding in social groups. That combination is a formula for creating more socially supportive groups.

We already saw this to a degree in the case of Maya. By focusing on involvement in a workers' union at the end of therapy, it gave her a place to put her greater emotional openness and the values-based motivation that was the flip side of her sense of unfairness.

The point is that intervention science has a great deal to contribute to positive psychology and cultural development in a wide range of areas, from racism to political healing, from immigration to climate change, from poverty to prosociality. Once the processes of change are clear, there is no reason to restrict clinical intervention science to buildings with glass doors. These processes belong in our homes and statehouses, in our streets and on our television screens. These processes belong in the lives of those we serve.

CHAPTER 13

Using the Tools of PBT in Practice

We want to conclude this book with a set of additional recommendations for how to build process-based therapy sensibilities and analytic tools into practical intervention work. Some of these specific topics and recommendations may not apply to you. PBT is a vast area, and while this book has been aimed primarily at mental health clinicians, the tools we have been describing can apply to any intervention practitioner—from life coaches to parent trainers, from child development specialists to gerontologists.

We should also note at the outset that a PBT approach is based on network thinking, but it is not synonymous with complex network analysis as such. We have emphasized the tools of network analysis in this book because it is one of the most powerful methods to foster process-based thinking, but the goal is the organized and dynamic use of processes of change, not a specific methodology.

Indeed, over time, experienced process-based therapists are able intuitively to build dynamical systems on the fly even without formally drawing out networks. In that regard it is worth recognizing that some of the practical tools you may have already been trained to deploy (traditional functional analysis, case conceptualization, the downward arrow technique in cognitive therapy, the Matrix in ACT, and so on) are actually mini-network tools that can be deployed as part of a larger PBT approach. These tools are too numerous for us to list here, but we encourage you to use these additional tools if they foster a process-based focus. We should not confuse any one particular tool with the essence of the approach itself, and as PBT evolves, we expect a rapid rise in assessment and analytic tools that have been shown to aid in PBT.

Speaking of tools, all of the diagrams in this book can easily be drawn using tools you likely have on your computer right now in the form of graphics or presentation programs. We drew the diagrams using a free online program called diagrams.net, and, having become skilled in its use, we can easily redraw entire networks in minutes.

Let's start with some recommendations for how best to make sure that network analysis is both doable and useful. You will not stick with a cumbersome method that does not improve outcomes, so a focus on efficiency and impact should be part of the learning process itself.

BUILDING NETWORKS WITH YOUR CLIENTS

Probably the single fastest way to make using network analysis easier, more relevant, and more time efficient is to build networks during session time with clients. Of course, not every client is appropriate for this approach, and you will need to learn how best to make it happen, but there are several major advantages of taking this approach.

For one thing, the nodes and edges in a PBT network should be empirical, not just conceptual. In the long run, that can best happen by using automated tools linked to repeated longitudinal assessment, but a quick way to begin is to rely on the client's actual experience. You can easily create networks right in session, being guided by the client and checking in as you go to see whether or not a diagram fits the client's experience. The arrows in network diagrams are just conditional probabilities—and the client will generally know a lot about what these conditional probabilities are in their experience if you ask in the right way. You should stay away from syndromal or other evaluative terms (such as "major depression" or "PTSD") and instead stick with more descriptive terms using the client's own language. We know from idiographic studies of client self-report that it is harder to compare frequency estimations across clients than within them. Fortunately, however, well-crafted networks rely more on consistency *within* the person about what is more or less dominant than consistency *across* people about what verbal estimates would translate to in observed actions. In deciding which arrows have larger or smaller arrow heads and which ones are single-headed or double-headed and so on, many if not most clients can do a relatively adequate job of saying what leads to what.

There are exceptions. Some clients have been so thoroughly dominated by DSM/ICD categories that they cannot describe their experience. They may also have lost a sense of their own autobiographical memory, inside a vague but painful label or state of mind (e.g., "I'm really depressed"). Thus, the advice to work with client estimates cannot be absolute, but when it is possible it can be very efficient.

The guiding questions in chapters 4, 5, and 6 can be helpful in this effort to dig down to a client's actual experience. Specific questions about what they're doing, how their life is unfolding, when things work, and when they don't will often reveal that the person actually has a lot of information they can use to understand and change variation and selection processes, but they're not doing it because they do not know where to look or how to formulate it. The average person does not look at their own life as a network or think about variation and selective retention in context linked to ways of being and doing. We do not need to try to teach such technical language—that is more for the therapist—but we can ask about what leads to what, when, and what then happens.

A major potential benefit of doing a network analysis collaboratively with clients is increasing the likelihood of achieving a common understanding. As the network takes shape, you can say things like:

- Does that look right?

- Does that fit your experience?

- Is there anything missing?

- Is there something we're emphasizing too much, or too little?

- What do you think? Is this really a double-headed relationship or is it more a one-way street?

You will get immediate feedback—and when it is worked out, you are more likely to have greater buy-in.

Doing network analyses in session also greatly reduces your time burden. When caseloads are high and time between clients is low, time can be of the essence. Doing networks in session can be extremely time efficient. Fortunately, it is more than that: you are also doing therapy even as you lay out the issues. Network analysis can be a powerful avenue to effectiveness.

The biggest impact of the working alliance in terms of positive outcomes is getting the client and you on the same page regarding what the issue is and what to do about it. The client is the expert in their own life, but they're not the expert in processes of change. As we bring in our knowledge of processes of change and fit that knowledge to the client's life as it is actually lived, we help the person see that they are not broken—rather that a system has ensnared them.

This collaborative effort can be therapeutic in and of itself. Seeing how mindless patterns serve unhelpful functions, for example, often itself removes or diminishes those unhelpful functions. For instance, knowing that you are avoiding something necessarily means that the avoidance is not complete, which can strengthen a new way forward.

CREATING A PBT SESSION NOTE SYSTEM

The issue of session notes raises another practical benefit of network analysis: it is not hard to write session notes linked to PBT strategies. Many systems of care want notes to be linked to outcomes, and the clarity of a process-based approach makes that relatively easy.

If the system of care demands a traditional psychiatric diagnosis, of course that will need to be provided. If the system demands a symptom focus, try to take notes using more observational terms (e.g., "depressed mood" instead of "depression"), but then focus on agreed-upon therapy goals with proximal process targets. For example, suppose a person is avoiding work because of anxiety. The process target may be greater emotional openness, as indicated by greater response flexibility and functionality in the presence of challenging emotions, including coming to therapy, being more able to examine and describe difficult emotions in session, being more willing to engage in exposure exercises, and decreasing work absences. Whatever system is in place (e.g., problem-oriented medical records, "SOAP" notes that describe subjective and objective data before an assessment and plan) can usually accommodate this kind of process-based focus.

By linking process targets to outcomes that are immediate, intermediate, and longer term, inclusion of outcomes in effect becomes an organizational process so that client processes of change become proximal outcomes. That same spirit can be used in session to hold yourself accountable to the client for outcome, which shifts the focus to processes.

A benefit of this approach is that ecological momentary assessment (EMA) data, periodic process measures, end-of-session measures, observation of in-session actions, and so on become all of a piece. Taking notes about the willingness of the person to, say, talk about difficult emotions in therapy without avoidance might be in the same bucket as seeking out life situations and learning to function well even if those situations will elicit those same difficult emotions. In essence, note-taking and formal and informal idiographic assessment become a way to track processes of change, held to account to outcome goals.

This approach will become more automated as repeated longitudinal assessment and EMA data become available via clinical support apps and the strength and structure of networks or subnetworks can be measured automatically. Tools of that kind are already emerging, but even before they become readily available, you can use the other tools we have described.

Of course, focusing on subnetworks has to be tempered by the place of this intervention in the larger set of relations. In this book we've emphasized that any process of change is part of an overall system. So you do need to periodically examine the overall network and take a peek at how things are changing.

SIMPLIFYING NETWORK MODELS

Human lives are complex. Think about what it would take to write an adequate biography of almost anyone you know well. It would likely take quite a substantial volume, and there would still be more to say.

Fortunately, clinical interventions are only part of an individual's life story. A complex network of a client is not a biography—it's a tool to get to the essence of what is important to make wise intervention choices and to track progress toward the accomplishment of agreed-upon goals.

If this purpose is loosened, networks can grow unreasonably. They can become excessively complex. Initially, you want a broad enough view that you have a holistic picture of the client's situation, tempered by the practical purpose of the exercise. An initially complex network is not a bad thing it if feels apt, but there is no need to use the idea of a "complete" network to push you toward excessive complexity. If anything really important is missing, it will tend to appear as you intervene.

The even more dominant pattern is that intervention focuses on particular areas, and the complex network is revisited only periodically and simplifies as treatment progresses. As subnetworks become the focus of treatment, for example, it is usually not hard to describe and track edges or subnetworks using only a sentence or two to summarize that aspect of the network. A two- or three-node network is easy to draw by hand and to use in session or to place in session notes.

Networks can be simplified in several ways. The best network is the simplest one that can accomplish the purposes of process-based functional analysis. The single most important purpose of all treatment utility is selecting and applying intervention in ways that maximize the probability of goal attainment. Other goals include being able to understand and describe the case, to track progress, and to gather knowledge that increases the progressivity of the field. In short, you are using these tools to help know what to do, and anything that can simplify treatment without reducing positive impact is helpful.

One simplifying strategy is to combine nodes of a network based on similar functions. Suppose a person is ruminating, worrying, and procrastinating. Initially these may be modeled as separate nodes, but if they are shown to have similar functions and to engage similar processes, a single node can list them all. For example, all three might be found to be features of perfectionism in a given client, perhaps driven by fear of social rejection. As functions become clearer, you may be able to simplify the network without practical cost.

Another avenue toward simplification is to include only information of practical importance given the purpose of intervention. This is similar to the classic idea in behavior therapy of an assessment funnel (Hawkins, 1979), which begins with a wide focus that narrows over time as the core issues become clearer. Likewise, as particular goals become more emphasized, minor goals and the events related to them can be dropped. Some of this may simply be driven by practical concerns. If an issue is unlikely to be targeted anytime soon and seems to be of marginal relevance to what is being treated, it can be dropped. Of course, these issues are not forgotten, and if their relevance becomes evident later on, they can be drawn back into the analysis.

A wonderful route into simplification may occur when issues are addressed so sufficiently that there is no particular reason to include them. In the case of Maya, for example, her rumination may settle down into a range that no longer needs to be tracked. In a case like that, remove it from the network. You don't need it in there anymore as a living clinical tool—it's not like you've forgotten it. You can reexamine the issue as part of termination planning.

Another source of simplification is theory. As you apply the EEMM to the network, and then apply measures to it, nodes and edges may recede in importance. When you realize they are not central, empirically and conceptually, drop them. Complexity without purpose is another name for distraction.

NOTING THE HIERARCHY OF PROCESSES

Some of the most important and studied processes of change extend across rows of the EEMM. Mindfulness is attentional but also affective and cognitive and touches on issues of self. Rumination and worry is attentional and cognitive and touches on issues of affect. Psychological flexibility cuts across all six psychological dimensions. And increasingly there are biophysiological dimensions being discovered that relate to such processes, and sociocultural extensions of them.

What this suggests is that as a PBT approach gathers strength, we may find more clustering of individual cases into functional analytic categories. It may soon be possible to link a case to a "process prototype" in which a characteristic network is nomothetically available that summarizes many idiographic networks and hierarchical processes that contain and organize more specific processes of change.

That day will be hastened by noting how processes of change nest themselves into hierarchical groupings. You can see the beginning of this in the way that retention and contextual sensitivity naturally emphasize some process dimensions over others.

For now, we will need to be finer grained because the empirical data are just not sufficient to know what these hierarchical arrangement and process prototypes will be. We have noticed that practitioners who use the network tools are creating and modifying them mentally on the fly. We are not yet to the point that most researchers can look at a network in an empirical study and know what it means. If we are right and the field is headed in an idiographically focused process-based direction, getting comfortable with thinking in this dynamic way will lead to major changes in research and practice.

SHARING NETWORKS WITH COLLEAGUES

As process-based thinking enters into clinics and systems of care, entire teams are now using process-based functional analysis in case conferences and network tools in case presentations. This is a wonderful thing, and we've found that a process-based focus quickly breaks down barriers between behavioral, cognitive, psychodynamic, systems, humanistic, and other perspectives.

We suggest that if you are in a theoretically diverse work team, you start with introducing processes of change as a focus but avoid fighting over terms. If a supervisor or higher administrator favors model or process focus X over your model or process focus Y, you may be able to assess both and to openly consider your case from both vantage points. Be catholic with a small c and let experience and data be the guide from there.

Once a process focus is familiar, try to explicate the functional, contextual spirit that's inside an extended evolutionary synthesis of variation, selection, retention, and context. You can begin by using more common-sense terms if evolutionary ones might be controversial (all practitioners talk in one way or another about healthy change, positive functions, maintaining gains, and being situationally sensitive). From there, a mini-network can help get the team thinking in a more precise way, and network analysis will be a natural next step.

The biggest resistance we have run into is not by those clinging to a particular theoretical orientation but by some who are hanging on to syndromes and protocols as the only way to do evidence-based therapy. For that wing of the audience, a focus on personalized medicine—of the need to fit empirical methods to the complexity of the individual—seems to be the best way to reduce needless resistance to the use of these methods.

Epilogue

We've come to the end of our journey together. We hope this book is helpful in enabling you to learn how to do process-based therapy. PBT is not a new form of therapy. It emerged from within the behavioral and cognitive tradition, but it applies in principle to any intervention approach for any population and from any theoretical orientation. PBT is a model of what evidence-based intervention even means. All approaches, disciplines, and methods focused on changing human functioning can play this game.

Our dominant focus in this book has been on psychotherapy, but the general approach could apply equally well to organizational change, or teaching, or occupational therapy, or applied behavior analysis with children with autism, and so on, through the entire list of human-focused applied behavioral disciplines.

We have lived far too long inside a failed diagnostic system that has biomedicalized human suffering. That approach has failed us and those we serve—and it is time to say so directly. The "protocols-for-syndromes" era has run its course, but it has left behind a vast body of knowledge on processes of change that can be retooled for a new, idiographic, functional, and contextual approach that avoids the ergodic error, breaks down the needless barriers between approaches, and draws researchers and practitioners into a more equal alliance that puts the client, clinical creativity, and scientific foundations back into better balance.

We're opening a new chapter of the story of intervention science and practice that has a chance to change how we do clinical work, but also to change our role in the culture. As we learn how to alleviate suffering *and* how to promote human prosperity, we become culturally relevant in a new and more powerful way. And as we learn how to deploy evidence-based treatment kernels in a person- and process-specific way, we exit the era of "one size fits all" and enter a new world in which the needs and background of the individual person *matter*.

The world needs knowledge like that. Now.

Science, technology, and rapid social change have stretched our ability to live in a balanced way. The modern world is a continuous challenge to human beings. As professionals, we need to support humanity in stepping forward into that new world in a new way, managing psychological challenges more compassionately and effectively. For that to happen we need a fundamental rethinking of what "evidence-based intervention" even is. No one can learn all of the protocols for all of the syndromal forms, but it may be quite possible to learn how to encourage ways of thinking, feeling, living, and relating that embody evidence-based processes of change and that apply to many life situations. It is fine to begin with the alleviation of a mental health problem, but intervention science and practice should not end there. Our clients want more from us; our communities and society need more from us. The existing data inside our research on psychological treatments forms a basis to do far more, but to make that journey we need a new vision and a new empirical agenda for the science of helping people change. We need to learn how to build and maintain processes of change that truly make a difference—healthy processes that empower healthy lives.

References

Barlow, D. H., Farchione, T. J., Fairholm, C. P., Ellard, K. K., Boisseau, C. L., Allen, L. B., & Ehrenreich-May, J. (2010). *Unified protocol for transdiagnostic treatment of emotional disorders: Therapist guide.* Oxford University Press.

Baron, R. M., & Kenny, D. A. (1986). The moderator-mediator variable distinction in social psychological research: Conceptual, strategic, and statistical considerations. *Journal of Personality and Social Psychology, 51*(6), 1173–1182. https://doi.org/10.1037/0022-3514.51.6.1173

Beard, C., Sawyer, A. T., & Hofmann, S. G. (2012). Efficacy of attention bias modification using threat and appetitive stimuli: A meta-analytic review. *Behavior Therapy, 43*(4), 724–40. https://doi.org/10.1016/j.beth.2012.01.002

Beck, A. T. (1976). *Cognitive therapy and the emotional disorders.* International Universities Press.

Border, R., Johnson, E. C., Evans, L. M., Andrew Smolen, A., Berley, N., Sullivan, P. F., & Keller, M. C. (2019). No support for historical candidate gene or candidate gene-by-interaction hypotheses for major depression across multiple large samples. *American Journal of Psychiatry, 176*(5), 376–387. https://doi.org/10.1176/appi.ajp.2018.18070881

Chase, J. A., Houmanfar, R., Hayes, S. C., Ward, T. A., Vilardaga, J. P., & Follette, V. M. (2013). Values are not just goals: Online ACT-based values training adds to goal-setting in improving undergraduate college student performance. *Journal of Contextual Behavioral Science, 2*(3–4), 79–84. http://doi.org/10.1016/j.jcbs.2013.08.002

Dawkins, R. (1976). *The selfish gene.* Oxford University Press.

Dobzhansky, T. (1973). Nothing in biology makes sense except in the light of evolution. *American Biology Teacher, 35*(3), 125–129. https://doi.org/10.2307/4444260

Gates, K. M., & Molenaar, P. C. M. (2012). Group search algorithm recovers effective connectivity maps for individuals in homogeneous and heterogeneous samples. *NeuroImage, 63*, 310–319.

Gifford, E. V., Kohlenberg, B., Hayes, S. C., Pierson, H., Piasecki, M., Antonuccio, D., & Palm, K. (2011). Does acceptance and relationship-focused behavior therapy contribute to bupropion outcomes? A randomized controlled trial of FAP and ACT for smoking cessation. *Behavior Therapy, 42*(4), 700–715. https://doi.org/10.1016/j.beth.2011.03.002

Hawkins, R. P. (1979). The functions of assessment: Implications for selection and development of devices for assessing repertoires in clinical, educational, and other settings. *Journal of Applied Behavior Analysis, 12*(4), 501–516. https://doi.org/10.1901/jaba.1979.12-501

Hayes, S. C. (2004). Acceptance and commitment therapy, relational frame theory, and the third wave of behavior therapy. *Behavior Therapy, 35*(4), 639–665. https://doi.org/10.1016/S0005-7894(04)80013-3

Hayes, S. C., & Hofmann, S. G. (Eds.) (2018). *Process-based CBT: The science and core clinical competencies of cognitive behavioral therapy.* New Harbinger Publications.

Hayes, S. C., & Hofmann, S. G. (2020). *Beyond the DSM: A process-based approach.* Context Press / New Harbinger Publications.

Hayes, S. C., Hofmann, S. G., Ciarrochi, J., Chin, F. T., & Baljinder, S. (2020, December). *How change happens: What the world's literature on the mediators of therapeutic change can teach us.* Invited address given to the Evolution of Psychotherapy Conference, Erickson Foundation.

Hayes, S. C., Hofmann, S. G., Stanton, C. E., Carpenter, J. K., Sanford, B. T., Curtiss, J. E., & Ciarrochi, J. (2019). The role of the individual in the coming era of process-based therapy. *Behaviour Research and Therapy, 117*, 40–53. https://doi.org/10.1016/j.brat.2018.10.005

Hayes, S. C., Hofmann, S. G., & Wilson, D. S. (in press). Clinical psychology is an applied evolutionary science. *Clinical Psychology Review.* https://doi.org/10.1016/j.cpr.2020.101892

Hayes, S. C., Strosahl, K. D., & Wilson, K G. (2016). *Acceptance and commitment therapy* (2nd ed.). Guilford Press.

Hesser, H., Westin, V., Hayes, S. C., & Andersson, G. (2009). Clients' in-session acceptance and cognitive defusion behaviors in acceptance-based treatment of tinnitus distress. *Behaviour Research and Therapy, 47*(6), 523–528. https://doi.org/10.1016/j.brat.2009.02.002

Hofmann, S. G. (2011). *An introduction to modern CBT: Psychological solutions to mental health problems.* Wiley-Blackwell.

Hofmann, S. G., Curtiss, J. E., & Hayes, S. C. (2020). Beyond linear mediation: Toward a dynamic network approach to study treatment processes. *Clinical Psychology Review, 76*, 101824. https://doi.org/10.1016/j.cpr.2020.101824

Hofmann, S. G., & Hayes, S. C. (2019). The future of intervention science: Process-based therapy. *Clinical Psychological Science, 7*(1), 37–50. https://doi.org/10.1177/2167702618772296

Insel, T., Cuthbert, B., Garvey, M., Heinssen, R., Pine, D. S., Quinn, K., Sanislow, C., & Wang, P. (2010). Research domain criteria (RDoC): Toward a new classification framework for research on mental disorders. *The American Journal of Psychiatry, 167*(7), 748–751. https://ajp.psychiatryonline.org/doi/full/10.1176/appi.ajp.2010.09091379

Kazantzis, N., Luong, H. K., Usatoff, A. S., Impala, T., Yew, R. Y., & Hofmann, S. G. (2018). The processes of cognitive behavioral therapy: A review of meta-analyses. *Cognitive Therapy and Research, 42*(5), 349–357. https://doi.org/10.1007/s10608-012-9476-1

Klepac, R. K., Ronan, G. F., Andrasik, F., Arnold, K. D., Belar, C. D., Berry, S. L., Christofff, K. A., Craighead, L. W., Dougher, M. J., Dowd, E. T., Herbert, J. D., McFarr, L. M., Rizvi, S. L., Sauer, E. M., & Strauman, T. J. (2012). Guidelines for cognitive behavioral training within doctoral psychology programs in the United States: Report of the Inter-Organizational Task Force on Cognitive and Behavioral Psychology Doctoral Education. *Behavior Therapy, 43*(4), 687–697. https://doi.org/10.1016/j.beth.2012.05.002

Levin, M. E., Hildebrandt, M. J., Lillis, J., & Hayes, S. C. (2012). The impact of treatment components suggested by the psychological flexibility model: A meta-analysis of laboratory-based component studies. *Behavior Therapy, 43*(4), 741–756. https://doi.org/10.1016/j.beth.2012.05.003

Olfson, M., & Marcus, S. C. (2010). National trends in outpatient psychotherapy. *American Journal of Psychiatry, 167*(12), 1456–1463. https://doi.org/10.1176/appi.ajp.2010.10040570

Paul, G. L. (1969). Behavior modification research: design and tactics. In C. M. Franks (Ed.), *Behavior therapy: Appraisal and status* (pp. 29–62). McGraw-Hill.

Probsta, T. Mühlbergerb, A., Kühner, J., Eifert, G., Pieh, C., Hackbarth, T., & Mander, J. (2020). Development and initial validation of a brief questionnaire on the patients' view of the in-session realization of the six core components of acceptance and commitment therapy. *Clinical Psychology in Europe, 2*(3), e3115. https://doi.org/10.32872/cpe.v2i3.3115

Tinbergen, N. (1963). On aims and methods of ethology. *Zeitschrift fuer Tierpsychologie, 20*(4), 410–433. https://doi.org/10.1111/j.1439-0310.1963.tb01161.x

Waddington, C. H. (1953a). Genetic assimilation of an acquired character. *Evolution, 7*, 118–126.

Waddington, C. H. (1953b). Epigenetics and evolution. *Symposia of the Society of Experimental Biology, 7*, 186–199.

Wegner, D. M. (1994). *White bears and other unwanted thoughts: Suppression, obsession, and the psychology of mental control.* Guilford Press.

Weisz, J. R., Chorpita, B. F., Palinkas, L. A., Schoenwald, S. K., Miranda, J., Bearman, S. K., Daleiden, E. L., Ugueto, A. M., Ho, A., Martin, J., Gray, J., Alleyne, A., Langer, D. A., Southam-Gerow, M. A., Gibbons, R. D., & the Research Network on Youth Mental Health. (2012). Testing standard and modular designs for psychotherapy treating depression, anxiety, and conduct problems in youth: A randomized effectiveness trial. *Archives of General Psychiatry, 69*(3), 274–282. https://doi.org/10.1001/archgenpsychiatry.2011.147

Stefan G. Hofmann, PhD, is Alexander von Humboldt Professor in the department of clinical psychology, Philipps-University Marburg, Marburg/Lahn, Germany; and professor of psychology in the department of psychological and brain sciences at Boston University. He has been president of numerous professional organizations, and is currently editor in chief of *Cognitive Therapy and Research*. He has published more than 500 scientific articles and twenty-five books. He is a highly cited researcher, and has received many awards, including the Humboldt Research Award. His research focuses on the mechanism of treatment change, translating discoveries from neuroscience into clinical applications, emotion regulation, and cultural expressions of psychopathology. He is codeveloper of process-based therapy (PBT) with Steven C. Hayes.

Steven C. Hayes, PhD, is Nevada Foundation Professor in the department of psychology at the University of Nevada, Reno. He has been president of numerous professional organizations, is author of forty-seven books and more than 650 scientific articles, and is among the most cited living psychologists. He has shown in his research how language and thought leads to human suffering, and is originator and codeveloper of acceptance and commitment therapy (ACT): a powerful therapy method that is useful in a wide variety of areas; relational frame theory (RFT): an empirical program in language and cognition; and PBT, with Stefan G. Hofmann.

David N. Lorscheid is a psychological coach and science writer. After completing his BSc in psychology at the Radboud University in Nijmegen, Netherlands, he specialized in helping people with low self-esteem and social anxiety. His business, Feel Confidence, uses evidence-based psychotherapy techniques in a fun and playful way to help people overcome their fears and become more confident. As of this point, his workshops and seminars have been attended by thousands of people from over twenty countries, and his articles have reached over one million readers.

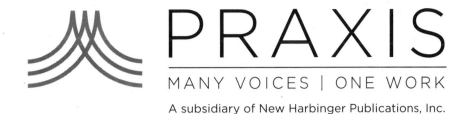

MORE BOOKS from
NEW HARBINGER PUBLICATIONS

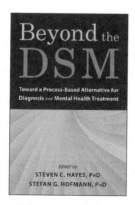
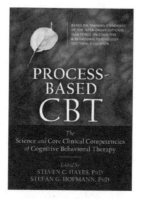
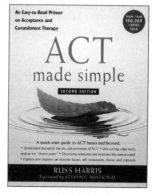
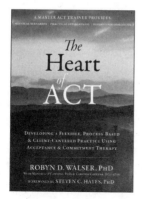
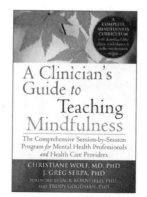
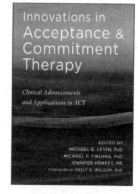

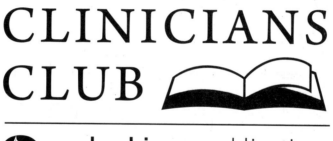

CLINICIANS CLUB

newharbingerpublications

Join the New Harbinger Clinicians Club—Exclusively for Mental Health Professionals

In our ongoing dedication to supporting you and your essential work with clients, we created the **New Harbinger Clinicians Club—** an entirely free membership club for mental health professionals.

Join and receive these exclusive club member benefits:

- A special welcome gift

- 35% off all professional books

- **Free client resources for your practice**—such as worksheets, exercises, and audio downloads

- **Free e-books throughout the year**

- **Access to private sales**

- A subscription to our *Quick Tips for Therapists* email program, new book release alerts, and e-newsletter

- **Free e-booklets of the most popular** *Quick Tips for Therapists*

- **Surveys on book topics you'd like to see us publish,** and resources you're looking for to better serve your clients

Join the New Harbinger Clinicians Club today at

newharbinger.com/clinicians-club

Did you know there are free tools you can download for this book?

Free tools are things like **worksheets, guided meditation exercises**, and **more** that will help you get the most out of your book.

You can download free tools for this book—whether you bought or borrowed it, in any format, from any source—from the **New Harbinger** website. All you need is a NewHarbinger.com account. Just use the URL provided in this book to view the free tools that are available for it. Then, click on the "download" button for the free tool you want, and follow the prompts that appear to log in to your NewHarbinger.com account and download the material.

You can also save the free tools for this book to your **Free Tools Library** so you can access them again anytime, just by logging in to your account! Just look for this button on the book's free tools page:

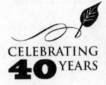

+ save this to my
free tools library

If you need help accessing or downloading free tools, visit **newharbinger.com/faq** or contact us at customerservice@newharbinger.com.

CELEBRATING
40 YEARS